Zany, Zeal, Zest and ZING

the Z Way to Happiness

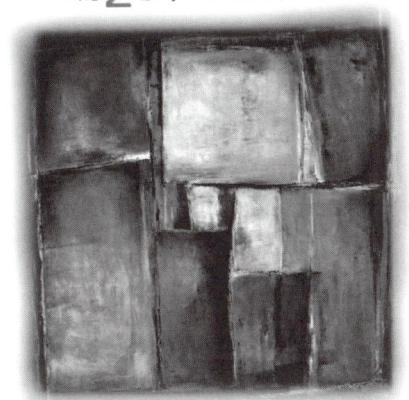

To Naeem and family.
With best wishes
for much happiness
always.

Shaila

Zany, Zeal, Zest and Zing
the Z Way to Happiness

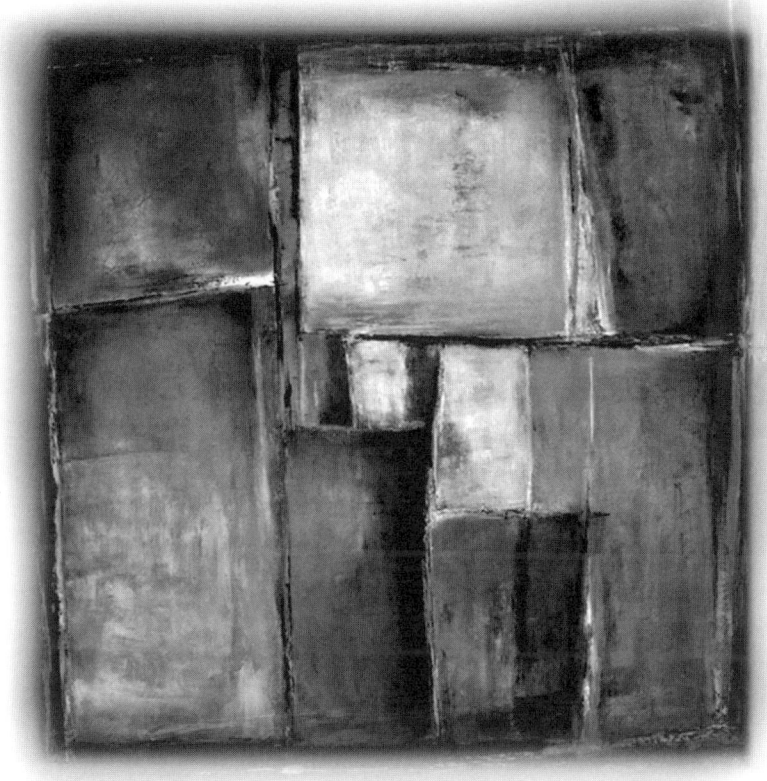

Zaibun
Ngee Ann Polytechnic, Singapore

World Scientific

NEW JERSEY · LONDON · SINGAPORE · BEIJING · SHANGHAI · HONG KONG · TAIPEI · CHENNAI

Published by

World Scientific Publishing Co. Pte. Ltd.

5 Toh Tuck Link, Singapore 596224

USA office: 27 Warren Street, Suite 401-402, Hackensack, NJ 07601

UK office: 57 Shelton Street, Covent Garden, London WC2H 9HE

British Library Cataloguing-in-Publication Data
A catalogue record for this book is available from the British Library.

Cover image: Provided by Anne Severyns (www.anneseveryns.com).

ISBN-13 978-981-279-350-8 (pbk)
ISBN-10 981-279-350-X (pbk)

Typeset by Stallion Press
Email: enquiries@stallionpress.com

Printed in Singapore by World Scientific Printers

*This book is dedicated to the people
who have made me happy, and in
particular to Paul Drayson, my husband*

ACKNOWLEDGEMENTS

It is a pleasure to thank several people whose encouragement, support and assistance were vital to the production of this book. They include the following:

The staff of the Ngee Ann Polytechnic library.

Lim Bee Ang, the Reference Manager of the Ngee Ann Polytechnic library for locating materials for me and her support.

The Staff of World Scientific Publishing Co Pte Ltd for their assistance and advice.

Ms. Sandhya of World Scientific Publishing Company, for her patience, enthusiasm and brilliant contributions as editor.

Yvonne Tan Hui Ling of World Scientific Publishing Co Pte Ltd for her insightful contributions and assistance as co-editor.

Anne Severyns, for allowing me to use her painting entitled, 'Happiness' for the front cover of the book. This cheerful, dynamic painting well reflects the Z way to Happiness.

The many people, with whom I have interacted over the years, who have taught me how to be and keep happy.

My friends and family members, in particular my mother, for their incredible support, encouragement and belief in me.

Paul Drayson, my husband, for his love and devotion, for giving me much joy and happiness and for being my best friend.

CONTENTS

INTRODUCTION

Why Happiness? Well, I decided to write this book to help people to be happy. So many people I know are busy with their careers and their families that they often forget to relax and have fun. Too often, they are caught up in the business of generating more income for themselves and their family members that they do not have the time to be happy. I have friends who are depressed and unhappy over certain issues and problems so much so they have sought medical attention for this.

After deciding on the subject, I thought about the structure and content for the book. As with my previous book, *Managing Oneself: Footprints to Success*, I chose to present the material in a pragmatic yet inspirational style. I opted to provide practical tips and strategies for people to implement. I decided that it would be necessary to provide a historical framework about the subject as so much has been written, researched and said about the subject. To enable people to understand why Happiness is important to them, I included a chapter on the benefits of being happy and the consequences of being unhappy.

As I read what different scholars and philosophers had to say about Happiness, it soon became clear to me that I could arrange the strategies for happiness under certain headlines namely Zany, Zeal, Zest and Zing.

Zany relates to play and all things fun while Zeal refers to devotion to a cause, ideal or goal. With Zest things would be exciting, enjoyable and interesting. Zing, in turn, will make us feel energetic, lively and vivacious. People who apply or cultivate the Z way to happiness will surely experience happiness.

The Z way to happiness is my suggested approach to attaining happiness. Practice the Z way to happiness and you will be contented, happy, energized and exciting. I have practised the examples and strategies proposed in the book and experienced much happiness for myself. Hence, I would like to share them with you so that you can experience happiness as I did.

Use the Z way to happiness...Be Zany; Apply Zeal; Have Zest and Put Zing into Your Life...Be Happy.

Chapter 1

HAPPINESS IS A SERIOUS MATTER

EARLY HISTORY

Asia

Happiness, defined as perpetual enjoyment of life, is a subject which has been much discussed through the ages. The study of happiness began in China, India and Greece more than 2,500 years ago, by thinkers like Confucius, Mencius, Buddha and Aristotle. Confucius was of the view that people should focus on relationships and the great virtue of humanity. He believed that learning about humanity would give us much joy. He argued that people have the power to transform themselves. Mencius preached that everyone has sprouts of virtue in them. If they extend these sprouts to social and political relationships, they will experience great joy. Mencius was of the view too that the more joy we experience in the process, the more motivated we become and the more we grow. Zhuangzi, a follower of Laozi, stressed the importance of a sense of humour and laughter. This is because it helps to release us from rationality and we can go along with things and then experience the oneness of the Dao. Buddha taught the eightfold path, the core of which involves the mind as a way to achieve happiness.

Greece and Rome

To the Greek Philosopher, Aristotle (384–322 BC) happiness meant being virtuous by choosing moderation in all things. He was of the view that all human beings want happiness. He said that *"happiness is the meaning and the purpose of life, the whole aim and end of human existence."* According to Aristotle, happiness is an activity. Happiness involves living the right way. To experience a happy life we need to have a sense of fulfillment. This means to have the feeling that we are doing something with our lives, and achieving something of ourselves. All this requires effort and commitment. This is why Aristotle described happiness as *"an activity of the soul."* Aristotle was of the view that happiness is a life-long pursuit.

Another Greek philosopher, Epicurus (342–270 BC) maintained that the key to happiness is pleasure. Pleasure should be the aim of every action and embracing it is especially good and healthy. He advocated the cultivation of simple and lasting pleasures. To Epicurus, **"pleasure is the beginning and end of living happily."** The ideals that he proposed were good wholesome food, the company of friends and a simple lifestyle. Seneca (4 BC–65 AD), a Roman, believed that the values of detachment and indifference could make him experience happiness in the most awful situations. We will, according to Seneca, enjoy ever lasting freedom and tranquility once we dismiss all that frightens and worries us. Epictetus (AD 55-135), a Greek philosopher, developed a philosophy that enabled him to endure slavery, disability and banishment cheerfully. He recognized that we cannot always control our circumstances, but we can control how we react to those circumstances. As he said, *"I must die. But must I die groaning? I must be imprisoned. But must I whine as well? I must suffer exile. Can anyone hinder me from going with a smile and a good courage, and at peace?"* According to Epictetus, we must accept the circumstances as they are for only then will we find Happiness. According to St. Augustine

4

(354–430 BC), happiness lies in the possession of an invaluable good, and this requires living a moral life.

18th and 19th Century

In 1776, Thomas Jefferson included *"the pursuit of happiness"* as a basic human right in the American Declaration of Independence. The Declaration promotes the right and responsibility of every person to pursue happiness. Happiness hence, is a work perpetually in progress. 18th Century thinkers like Jeremy Bentham argued that the best society is that where the people are happiest and the best policy is the one that produces the greatest happiness. Bentham believed that happiness was equal to pleasure and he stated that a happy life is one in which pleasure outweighs pain. The Prussian philosopher, Immanuel Kant (1724–1804) emphasized that people should make themselves happy. He also said that *"morality is not properly the doctrine of how we make ourselves happy, but how we may make ourselves worthy of happiness."* According to the German philosopher, Arthur Schopenhauer (1788–1860), life can be improved through ascetic living, an appreciation of art and charity for one's fellow-men or loving kindness as he described it. He maintained that the two enemies of human happiness are *"pain and boredom."* John Stuart Mills (1806–1873), a British philosopher was of the view that some pleasures are more valuable than others. He separated pleasures into *"lower"* and *"higher"* ones. Lower pleasures include things like eating and drinking and these can be enjoyed by humans and animals alike. The higher ones include friendship, achievement, art, music and poetry. These can only be achieved by humans. Mills maintained that it is only when we pursue the higher pleasures that we can be happy and fulfilled.

20th Century

> "But what is happiness except the simple
> harmony between a person
> and the life they lead."

Albert Camus

The British philosopher, Bertrand Russell (1872–1970) was of the view that happiness is something that can be attained through hard work. He believed that *"a world full of happiness is not beyond human power to create."* Bertrand Russell explained that *"the real obstacles lie in the heart of man, and the cure for these is a firm hope."* Abraham Maslow was one of the first psychologists to examine the issue of happy people. He theorized that once the needs for food, security, love and self-esteem are satisfied, a deep desire for creative expression and self-actualization comes to the surface. Other psychologists like Carl Jung and Erich Fromm maintain that the desire for happiness demands attention. Mihaly Csikszentmihalyi believes that happiness does not just happen. It has to be planned for and worked at by setting challenges that are appropriate to one's abilities. The Dalai Lama wrote in his book, *The Art of Happiness* that the very purpose of life is to be happy. The Dalai Lama is of the view that the more we care for the happiness of others, the greater will be our sense of well-being. Mahatma Gandhi defined happiness as *"when what you think, what you say, and what you do are in harmony."* According to Ellen Keller, a clinical psychologist, *"happiness is a long lasting enduring enjoyment of life; it is being in love with living. It is your reward for achieving a good character and personal rational values in life."* The values which Ellen Keller considers important are a productive career, romance, friendship and hobbies. The writer, David Leonhart maintains that *"you don't find happiness, you make happiness."* Hence, some effort is required to achieve happiness. One needs to apply talents and abilities in the pursuit of happiness.

According to Ed Diener, a psychologist, *"philosophers considered happiness to be the highest good and ultimate motivation for human action."* Some will conclude that the purpose of life then is happiness. In Singapore, the word happiness appears in the Pledge which is taken by all citizens. The Pledge reads as follows: *"We, the citizens of Singapore pledge ourselves as one united people regardless of race, language or religion, to build a democratic society based on justice and equality, so as to achieve happiness, prosperity and progress for our nation."* Norman Bradburn in 1969 described happiness as having more positive emotions and moods than negative emotions and moods. Martin Seligman outlines three categories of positive emotions. These are:

- Past: feelings of satisfaction, contentment, pride, and serenity,
- Present (examples): enjoying the taste of food, glee at listening to music, absorption in reading, and
- Future: feelings of optimism, hope, trust, faith and confidence.

From his research, Martin Seligman concluded that there are three dimensions to happiness that can be cultivated. These are the *Pleasant Life*, the *Good Life* and the *Meaningful Life*. With the *Pleasant Life* the individual appreciates basic pleasures such as companionship, the natural environment and bodily needs. We experience the *Good Life* when we discover our virtues and strengths and use them to improve our lives. In the *Meaningful Life*, we apply our unique strengths for a greater purpose.

In 1976, Angus Campbell concluded that happiness included being satisfied with one's basic circumstances. In his book, *Happiness: Lessons from a New Science*, Lord Richard Layard defines *"happiness as feeling good — enjoying life and wanting the feeling to be maintained."* Other writers have defined happiness as how much a person appreciates the life he or she leads. To Matthieu Ricard, Happiness is *"a deep sense of flourishing that arises from an exceptionally healthy mind."* He views happiness as *"a way of interpreting the world"* and he maintains that *"while it may be difficult to change the world, it is always possible to change the way we look at it."* From these definitions and statements, we may conclude that there are many elements in the happiness formulae.

In an article written for the International Network on Personal Meaning, the President of the Network, Paul T.P. Wong stated that "a perfect picture of happiness is something like the sum total of the following elements:

- Moments of pleasure and enjoyment
- Positive feelings and thoughts
- Absence of negative feelings and thoughts
- Fully healthy and functioning
- Positive relationships
- Positive expectations of the future
- Positive actions
- Success and achievement
- Positive self-concept
- Positive assessment of one's life
- Virtues and strengths
- True love and good sex
- Humour and laughter
- Meaning and purpose"

THE ECONOMIC COST OF HAPPINESS

Despite huge increases in living standards, over the last fifty years, average happiness has not increased in Britain or in the USA. A 2006 study by the British think-tank New Economics Foundation (NEF), the Happy Planet Index, ranked Britain as

108th and the USA as 150th of a list of 178 nations. Singapore was ranked 131st. Vietnam was the best amongst the countries in the ASEAN region as it was ranked 12th. It would seem that some people who do not have much are very happy while others who seem to have much are not. According to researchers, the correlation between wealth and well-being is weak in affluent countries. Any additional income that they receive after being able to afford the necessities of life will only result in diminishing returns.

Is it true to say that governments have succeeded in delivering greater and greater wealth but that has not translated into extra happiness? Is seeking happiness only by improving material conditions the right approach to adopt? Should governments consider other approaches to generating happiness? Many research studies have also proven that money, fame and worldly success do not necessarily lead to happy and fulfilled lives. Lord Richard Layard argued that people who experience incapacitating bouts of depression and such states of unhappiness decrease the productivity of the whole society. Nations should help people to be happy.

POLITICAL RESPONSES TO THE HAPPINESS ISSUE

> "The aggregate happiness of society which is best promoted by the practice of a virtuous policy, is, or ought to be, the end of all government."

> George Washington

In 2002, the office of the British Prime Minister, Tony Blair published a paper which considered how happiness might affect different policies. The following were included in the paper:

- A happiness index
- Teaching people about happiness

- More support for volunteering
- A more leisured work-life balance
- Higher taxes for the rich

One generation ago, the monarch of Bhutan insisted that gross national happiness is more important than gross national product. The present Conservative leader in Britain, David Cameron believes that improving people's happiness is a key challenge for politicians. He maintains that politicians should not just make people better off but that they should make people happier, make communities more stable and make society more cohesive. He told The Happiness Formula programme: ***"We should be thinking not just what is good for putting money in people's pockets but what is good for putting joy in people's hearts."*** Indeed, if governments want people to be happier, they have to understand the conditions which bring happiness and implement measures to cultivate happiness in a society.

In Singapore, the government introduced a campaign in September 2007, "Healthy Mind, Happy Life" focusing on mental wellbeing. In its press release, the Singapore Health Promotion Board explained that the focus on mental wellbeing is in line with increasing global focus on this issue. In 2005, the World Health Organization (WHO) identified the promotion of mental wellbeing as important. It emphasized that with mental wellbeing, one in better able to realize one's own abilities, cope with the normal stresses of life, work productively and contribute to the community.

Lord Layard maintains that governments should include the happiness of its citizens at the heart of its public and economic policy. They should make work life more compatible with family life, reduce rates of mental illness and eliminate high unemployment. Another British economist, Andrew Oswald has proposed that achieving a proper work-life balance will contribute to the overall happiness in a country. One thing that we can be sure of is that wanting happiness for others is a positive, moral religious good.

"No matter how dull, or how mean, or how wise a man is, he feels that happiness is his indisputable right."

Helen Keller

SHOULD HAPPINESS BE TAUGHT?

At Harvard University in the United States of America and Cambridge University in Britain, courses on well-being and happiness are being offered. In England, at secondary level, Wellington College has introduced a course on happiness for its students with the purpose of producing young men and women who are happy and who know themselves and what they want to do in life. Through the happiness programme, the College aims to develop its students into people who are respected colleagues, valued friends and loving parents whose children will grow up in a secure environment in which they know they are valued and treasured.

Schools are the best place to teach happiness. This is because character and habits are in their formative stages in young people. It is much more difficult to acquire good habits later in life.

The course, as described by Dr Anthony Seldon, the Master of Wellington College, concentrates on emotional learning and emotional intelligence. It focuses on the development of personal responsibility. Dr Seldon believes that people **"can be taught emotional resilience, self-control, the habits of optimism, handling negative thoughts and much else."** The course provides students with the opportunity of learning how to manage their own bodies, minds and emotions, how to make the right decision and how to manage themselves when they feel lonely. The students learn about forming healthy and sustaining relationships. They learn how to identify and treasure good relationships and avoid relationships which are damaging and destructive. They will also gain an understanding about the goals they should want to establish in life. The happiness course at Wellington College will enable the students to learn more about themselves which they can put to use for the rest of their lives. Such a course, according to Dr Seldon would help people cope with personal difficulties in the future. These difficulties might include professional rejections, breakdown of relationships, bereavements and periods of depressions.

If happiness is not formally taught in schools, then information on happiness should be made easily available so that people can learn how to be happy.

Chapter 2

WHAT IS HAPPINESS?

A DESCRIPTION OF HAPPINESS

Happiness can be described as a long-term emotional state of being happy. It has also been defined as a positive, enduring state that consists of positive feelings and includes both peace of mind and active pleasures, elation and joy. It is a deep sense of engagement. Happy people feel life deeply. Happiness is described by some as a feeling of contentment created when all of one's physical, emotional, psychological, intellectual and spiritual needs have been gratified. It is really a long-term, inner feeling. When you are happy, you experience a feeling of great pleasure and a profound enduring sense of contentment and capability. Other emotions associated with happiness are joy, exultation, delight, bliss and love.

Happiness is a state of mind where a person feels that life is good. You live in the moment and you have great pleasure in all the treasures, in all the beautiful things that life has to offer. You experience an excellent quality of well-being; one that is generated from the recognition that you can effectively and creatively manage everything that life has to offer. You would, when happy, understand your internal self and react to your needs rather than what others wish of you. It is widely recognized today that happiness is much sought after by everyone and that it is indeed what makes our lives worthwhile.

ACHIEVING HAPPINESS

Can happiness be achieved without us giving what it takes to achieve it? Is true happiness the result of giving and not receiving? To find happiness we will need to be aware that disciplined determination on our part is required to achieve it. It is within our own power, our own strength and our own energy to find happiness. We can all make the best life possible for ourselves. We can all choose to be happy and avoid harbouring negative thoughts. Our attitude towards life, others and ourselves will affect our happiness. It is important that we appreciate what we have in life. We live in good homes. We love our work and we are healthy. We also have many friends and family members who provide us with much support and love.

Happiness does not come by occasionally. It is possible to increase our level of happiness by various methods. To achieve happiness, we have to work at it. It is a skill which must be learned. People are often unhappy because they are ignorant about the nature of happiness. We may also fail to recognize the value of happiness and the benefits of being happy. It helps therefore to read about happiness and to attend talks and courses on happiness. As **Jean- Jacques Rousseau** said, **"every man wants to be happy, but in order to be so he needs first to understand what happiness is."** We also learn about happiness through examples, rewards, stories, from the media and other sources.

THE CONSEQUENCES OF BEING UNHAPPY

On a Personal Level

> *"If one lets fear or hate or anger take possession of the mind, they become self-forged chains."*

> Helen Gallagher Douglas

14

We cannot be in a state of happiness if we experience unpleasant emotions. These emotions might be apathy, anger, annoyance, anxiety, boredom, depression, discontent, discouragement, dissatisfaction, envy, fear, frustration, grief, guilt, hatred, irritation, jealousy, sadness, shame, stress and worry. Fear, for example can generate cruelty and superstition. When we are unhappy, we are more prone to performing unpleasant and morally incorrect acts on ourselves and others. When we are unhappy, we affect others and make their lives unhappy too. If we are not at ease with ourselves, we cannot be at ease with others. We therefore have an obligation to be happy.

A happy person is therefore fundamental to the development of a happy society. To help the people around us, we should make it a point to be as happy as possible. When we are happy, we become better people. We cannot be happy and at peace if we are frustrated and disappointed. Hence, it is important that we understand what happiness is and what we can do to cultivate happiness. To be happy, we should eradicate the causes of unhappiness from our life. Some possible causes might be envy, relationship problems, loneliness and fear of the opinion of others.

On a Global Level

Unhappiness can not only affect our personal lives but also result in global problems. Wars and terrorism are brought about by people who are unhappy. When a country is not happy with certain issues, it may wage a war against another country. Terrorists who hurt others and attack people are not happy with issues and causes. These could be political, social, religious or economic issues. If a person were truly happy, he or she would not perform an act of terrorism on others. Unhappy people demonstrate a lack of respect and tolerance for other people, views and beliefs. Happiness in people results in a safer, less violent world for everyone.

THE BENEFITS OF BEING HAPPY

There are many advantages to being happy. A happy life is no doubt a better life to lead.

Health

> *"The joyfulness of a man prolongeth his days."*
>
> Sirach 30:22

Happy people get along well with others and live healthier lives. They are healthier both mentally and physically. There seems to be a strong correlation between happiness and biological fitness. Happy people exhibit better health habits, experience lower blood pressure and have a better immune system. They are much less likely to fall ill and they live longer, perhaps five to nine years longer. They generally take more health and safety precautions than other people. This might explain why they recover from sickness quicker. When you are happy, you are protected against many of the problems and negative effects of aging. Happy people cope with pain better than others. Happy people are less likely to develop problems with drugs and alcohol.

More Fulfilled

People who are happy are energetic and ambitious. They are also more vital and active. They always seem to have much to do and not enough time to do everything that they want to do. Happy people have a more positive outlook towards life and they consider the world to be safer. They tend to have favourable perceptions of the future and are more satisfied with life.

Happy people are fulfilled people. They also tend to be at peace with themselves and with their surroundings. They are less likely to commit crimes. When you are happy with yourself, you are less likely to be misunderstood. You are also less self-focused.

Relationships

Happy people have better relationships with others and are popular. They share their happiness with others, are considerate to people around them and are always willing to help others. Happy people are more likely to be more cooperative, prosocial and charitable. They make better friends. They experience fun-filled, long and fruitful marriages. Having better friendships and relationships between men and women in terms of marriage will make a difference to a society's happiness. Productive relationships with other people help to maintain the well-being of a society.

When we care for others we are less prone to depression. We should learn to be considerate to others and be happy because when we are unhappy and negative, we upset others. Happy people can respond to difficult people much better and are to forgive others. They are more satisfied with their friends and less jealous of others. Having good relationships generates happiness. Good relationships require responsibility, care, concern and dealing with burdens. When we give others our love and in return, are loved by them, we will enjoy happiness. Happy people are more likely to enjoy stronger social support and richer social interactions.

SENSE OF WELL-BEING

When we are happy, we enjoy a great sense of well being and express positive moods and emotions most of the time. In turn we engage in great thoughts, wisdom, intelligence and common sense. Happy people are more likely to be emotionally healthy. When we experience positive emotions we develop friendships, generate love, enjoy excellent physical health and experience greater achievement in our careers and lives. We are able to enhance our resources and develop our skills for the future. With happiness, we tend to respect ourselves and others as well. Happy people have higher self-esteem and appear more attractive to others.

Handle Emotions

People who are happy are better prepared to handle anger. They can also cope with fear, self-doubt, anxiety and despair. It is generally agreed that a happy person is a caring and concerned person. Happy people have ambitions and have been described by researchers as being more psychologically resilient, assertive, empathetic and open to experience.

Some other attributes and factors that help people to be happy are connectedness, social and emotional competence, communication skills, meaningful activity, a sense of control, resilience, optimism, and playfulness. Happiness enables us to better control our emotions. Happy people are compassionate, creative, and emotionally and physically healthy.

FACE CHALLENGES

"The days that make us happy make us wise."

John Masefield

Being happy enables us to do things that make us comfortable. We will be able to undertake tasks and find solutions to problems. Happy people have greater self-control and can

18

cope with challenges more effectively. When you are happy you feel that you can bring about many changes. You feel that you can cope with challenges that come your way. You are empowered to do things which you thought you could not handle. You will be able to function as a human being effectively if and when you are happy. To be happy, you need to live a life of purpose, to love and give as you try to realize your dreams.

Happiness is essential as it gives us a purpose for living and keeps us going even as we face challenges and problems. It is useful as it gives us something to look forward to and provides us hope. Happiness enables us to experience the best that life has to offer. With happiness we open up to the fullest for life, for challenges and opportunities. It is indeed an essential and important foundation for success.

WHY WE NEED HAPPY PEOPLE AT THE WORKPLACE

Happy workers are more productive. They produce better products because they are committed to their work and take pride in what they do. Another reason why we need happy people at the workplace is that they tend to be healthier. They are less likely to catch colds and recover from illness and accidents faster than an average person. Hence, organizations with happy people enjoy reduced absenteeism and medical leave. When employees are happy and like their work, they tend to be energetic. As a result, they cope with much more work than other employees. They excite others about work and encourage them to be more energetic as well. Happy, satisfied workers are less likely to suffer from job burnout and retaliatory behaviour.

In any workplace, communication is very important. One factor for success in the organization is good and effective communication. This can be achieved if employees are happy. Happy people generally communicate more openly and effectively with others. This enhances creativity within the organization. Happy employees experience lower levels of stress and anxiety, hence, they are less confused and can think more clearly. They can focus on their work and enjoy better concentration. Happy employees are better able to handle problems and can make decisions. When people are happy, they attend to their work more effectively and can perform their tasks better. Happy employees are generally more organized and efficient in their work.

Happy employees in an organization work well with each other. There is better teamwork and cooperation amongst the employees when they are happy. When people are happy working with each other, the organization experiences less employee turnover. Happy employees also enjoy job satisfaction and will do more than what is required of their job. They spread goodwill throughout the organization. They also react well with their clients and members of the public. A happy employee communicates effectively with clients and is able to reach out to clients in a courteous and friendly manner. Happy employees adopt a pleasant tone of voice and generate warmth. This makes clients happy. In turn, service quality will be enhanced. Sales will be increased. This should result in higher profits for the organization.

When employees are happy, they become more committed to their work and organization. They will work for the good of the organization and will help realize its strategic initiatives, values, vision and mission. The morale within the organization will improve. Supervision of staff in an organization is easier when the employees are happy and committed to their work. Employees in turn will enrich the organization with greater output. If employees are happy at work, they will leave their workplaces feeling happy. They will be in a happy frame of mind when they return home and they will remain happy.

BEING HAPPY HELPS

When you are happy, you can take action, you can make changes, do what you can and when you can. You can also find solutions to problems and be pro-active. You feel responsible. You take charge and can engage in activities that you probably thought you could not do. When we are happy, we are also able to make good choices.

YOU GENERATE YOUR OWN HAPPINESS

Our happiness or unhappiness is not the result of external causes, circumstances or actions by other people. No one can make us feel unhappy. We have the power within us to develop our own happiness. Henry David Thoreau said, *"There is no value in life except what you choose to place upon it and no happiness in any place except what you bring to it yourself."* Happy people are aware that they are able to control their situation. As happiness is a state of mind that is generated from within us, we can use our minds and intelligence to achieve happiness.

CHOOSE TO BE HAPPY

We can choose to be happy or unhappy. Indeed we have the choice. We must recognize that we are responsible for charting our own happiness. This is because we are in charge of our own lives and can decide on what is best for us. We have the relevant skills and knowledge to do so. We can develop attitudes that will encourage us not to feel unhappy. One's happiness then is affected by self-esteem, optimism, a sense of belonging and the capacity to love.

TAKE THE FIRST STEP

"If we are ever to enjoy life, now is the time — not tomorrow or next year. The best preparation for a better life next year is a full, complete, harmonious, joyous life this year."

Thomas Drier

Happiness is something that we can work at and this can be learnt. Acquisition of happiness should be a success goal. We have to invest serious effort to achieve real happiness. If we think that we are not in control of our lives, that we are controlled by others, then we will be depressed. When we take charge of our life and when we become responsible for ourselves, we will be happy. Avoid wasting time and energy worrying.

Choose to be happy. Each day tell yourself that you have the choice to be happy or not to be happy and you choose to be happy. Make an affirmation to yourself each day, "I feel happy and joyful today." Life is great. Happiness is to be found now and not in the distant future. So live it now. Right now is the best time to be happy. Enjoy it. Reach for it. Start to be happy. Be willing to be happy now. As you take that first step, you will experience a sense of boldness which will be magical for you. Look at each day as a new beginning with happiness ahead for you. You should treasure every moment that brings you happiness.

Chapter 3

BE ZANY

"Humour is the great thing, the saving thing. The minute it crops up, all our irritations and resentments slip away, and a sunny spirit takes their place."

Mark Twain

WHY BE ZANY?

To be zany is to be eccentric, bizarre, play the fool. Being zany helps us to be happy. We need to look for fun-filled experiences, to have fun and laugh every day. We need to have a good time as this is refreshing. Bertrand Russell maintained that we should do things for pleasure, things which have nothing to do with our work or responsibilities. If all that we do is to concentrate on our work and responsibilities, we will develop stress and worries and we will lack enthusiasm for anything else. When we undertake activities for fun we become energized and we feel relaxed. Cultivating other interests besides work, we soon realize that there is much going on outside of our own little sphere. When you have fun doing other things besides work, you will be happy and relaxed.

We feel exhilarated when we throw our heads back and have a hearty laugh and when we have a good time. So forget your inhibitions and act happy at all times. This will help you to be happier with yourself, with others and with life as a whole. Remember that no one can make us happy except ourselves. We can put ourselves into a particular frame of mind by the way we act. When we project a smiling expression, not only we but others too will feel good. You will feel happy if you talk as if you feel positive self-esteem and are optimistic.

BE WITH HAPPY AND FUN PEOPLE

To live a happy and healthy life, we need to be with fun people who can make us laugh. This should apply to our workplace, personal lives, and community work. Look for people with a sense of humour and an interesting insight on life. At all times, surround yourself with happy people. Happiness from others, be it a member of our family, a friend, a colleague, a neighbour or an acquaintance is contagious.

> *"Mirth is like a flash of lightning,that breaks through a gloom of clouds, and glitters for a moment; cheerfulness keeps up a kind of daylight in the mind, and fills it with a steady and perpetual serenity."*
>
> Joseph Addison

We have to learn how to laugh at ourselves and not to take ourselves too seriously. If you can engage in humour as often as possible, you will feel happy. Humour will help to make situations which are unbearable seem bearable. It will make a miserable outlook cheerful. Humour will help to improve situations at the workplace and make relationships seem fun and enjoyable.

BE A FUN PERSON

> *"Celebrate your success and find humour in your failures. Don't take yourself so seriously. Loosen up and everyone*

around you will loosen up. Have fun and always show enthu-siasm. When all else fails, put on a costume and sing a silly song."

Sam Walton

We need to be fun people ourselves. Remind yourself to have fun. To be fun people, we need to be inviting, interesting, open and expansive. We should reach out to others and build good relationships. Get to know as many people as possible. The old adage **"No man is an island unto himself"** is very true. We all need contact with others. Not only should we make contact with people but also develop productive relationships as these are crucial to maintaining our well-being. Happy people tend to give more of themselves and their time in relationships with other people. This means caring about other people. Be excited about other people, their lives, the work they do and the way they live their lives.

MAKE OTHERS HAPPY

We find happiness ourselves when we make others happy. Visit someone who is ill or suffering and when you see the person brighten up on seeing you, you too will feel better. It has been said that caring for others is a powerful antidote for depres-sion. When you receive excellent service at a restaurant, bar, beautician or hairdresser, leave a tip and make the person feel happy. In return, you too will receive good service each time you return to the same establishment. This will make you feel happy.

TIME IS PRECIOUS

We should recognize that each day, each hour and each minute is precious. We should savour every moment and enjoy every minute. We should not ponder about the past or live in the

25

future. We should just get on with life. Enjoy your life and what it offers you. Don't just sit around waiting for things to happen. Plan each day to ensure that you are fully occupied. Use your time cleverly and usefully. Immerse and absorb yourself in your work, love, friendship and leisure. Reach out, create events and have a positive impact on people, places and the world as a whole. As Luci Swindoll said, *"to experience happiness we must train ourselves to live in this moment, to savor it for what it is, not running ahead in anticipation of some future date nor lagging behind in the paralysis of the past."* Identify your strengths and virtues and use them more often in your life. You could also try using one of your strengths in a new way.

LOOK AT LIFE THROUGH THE EYES OF A CHILD

Zany people look at life through the eyes of a child. Everything is new, fun, and joyous. Be excited about life. Look at life as if it is one big adventure. Be a stimulant. We should live life, have fun and be happy. Each morning when you wake up, look forward to the day. Each day brings with it new challenges and plenty of potential. We need to keep busy, seek stimulation and novelty all the time. We should involve ourselves in new experiences and cultivate new interests. Invest your energies in things which have not been discovered. Try different, new and novel ways, and take courses which others have not explored. Experiment too with unusual and untried ways. This should make you a better person.

DO THE UNEXPECTED

Add sparkle to your life by doing the unexpected. Resist doing the routine and instead have something different from time to time. Be flexible with your time and energy. Here are some suggestions of things that you can do:

- Surprise someone with an unexpected gift.
- Have a meal with your spouse at a different place and time.
- Take a cruise to an exotic location.
- Invite someone over for an impromptu meal.
- Write to someone you have not been in touch with for awhile.
- Send notes of encouragement and appreciation to the people you know.
- When someone you know has experienced success, do not hesitate to celebrate this with them.
- Remember birthdays and anniversaries.
- Give your friends beautifully wrapped presents.
- Go for a walk or meet someone for a drink.
- Arrange an evening out with friends.
- Celebrate with champagne or wine.
- Cultivate interesting hobbies.
- If you feel like dancing on tables or on the bar top, just do it.
- Let your hair down.
- Take off your shoes and walk barefoot on the beach, on the road, on the grass or at home. Feel the grass under your feet.
- Enjoy the warmth of the sun on your face when you are outdoors.
- If you feel like colouring your hair purple, just do it. Don't wait till you are seventy five and then look back and regret what you have not done.
- Ride a roller coaster or on a merry go round.
- See a funny movie.

Create time for fun in your life. Incorporate in your daily schedule some time for fun. Allot time to engage in activities that you enjoy and to perform acts of silliness. Select one afternoon to act silly. When we do so, we are more likely to be happy and joyous. We will also feel as if we are someone else, a new person.

PLAY

Play as much as you can. Creative people play a great deal. In history, we note that the great artists, sculptors, scientists and philosophers engaged in play extensively — e.g. Picasso, Einstein and Jean-Paul Sartre. Play helped them discover ideas, art and adventure. When we play, we forget about ourselves and our childhood and adulthood merge into one. Play and be silly once in a while. Have fun with your friends by playing a prank on them. This will make you feel joyous. Leave a cheerful, fun-filled message and greetings for your friends on their voice mail. Do the bird dance or the hokey cokey. This is guaranteed to make you laugh and be happy.

We can play and have fun in virtually every activity in life. Try to have fun while you are working on something important and you will experience much happiness. Important activities in life might include bringing up children, developing your career and undertaking community service. If you need to fill up your time, apply for a fun, part-time job. Plan and organize a fun event once in a while. Just planning for it and going through the ideas for it in your mind will make you feel happy. A good event to organize is a block or street party as it will give you an opportunity to get to know your neighbours better. Plan an elegant dinner party. Immersing yourself in the details of this party will stimulate you and make you feel delighted.

SMILE

"Every time you smile at someone, it's an action of love,
A gift to that person, a beautiful thing."

Mother Theresa

Learn to smile more often. Try smiling as soon as you wake up in the morning. Smile as much as you can throughout each day. Smiling will make you look more pleasant and attractive. Happy people have pleasant expressions; so keep smiling so that you can maintain a pleasant expression at all times. Smiling can also change your mood and attitude. When we smile we communicate our happiness to others. This will encourage people to feel happy with us. Smile at a stranger along the corridor, on the street, at the lift, in the office and elsewhere. It might be the one happy moment in that person's day. A smile can work magic not just on others but on us too. Both the sender and the receiver of the smile will be inspired to be happy.

WHY SHOULD YOU SMILE?

Smiling has a positive effect. It makes you feel better and affects others positively as well. Occasionally, just look up and smile. Research has proven that we feel happier when we smile. It is definitely far better to smile than to frown or refrain from an expression. If you are smiling, people will react well to you. It sets the stage for a pleasant conversation with someone. When we smile at others, they will feel happy and good towards us. This, in turn, will make us feel happy. Find excuses to smile. Give a heartfelt smile always. Your smile will evoke smiles in others. Help others to smile and you will smile even more. Giving small gifts to others will make them smile. You will then feel happy. Joe Kapp, a footballer said, *"wake up with a smile and go after life…live it, enjoy it, taste it, smell it, feel it."*

WHAT YOU SHOULD DO

Try smiling even when you do not feel like doing so. You will find that whatever misery you may have will be soon dissipated and your personal happiness will develop. Practice smiling at people. Undertake small smiling exercises throughout the day. Smiling will help make our interactions with other people truly satisfying. A smile has been described as probably the most common symbol of happiness in people. We should try smiling throughout the day as it will help us to feel happy. It will also remind us that we should work towards being happy all the time. We will find our world less intimidating.

According to the August 2002 edition of *SHE Magazine*, researchers have identified at least 18 different types of smiles expressing all sorts of good emotions — happiness, enjoyment, pleasure, pride, relief and amusement. Happy people smile often, so cultivate the habit of smiling.

LAUGHTER

"Laughter is the most powerful state of mind there is. When you're laughing, you can't think of anything else."

H. Jackson Brown

Much has been written about laughter. Some writers who have written on this topic include Aristotle, Plato, Hobbes, Freud, Kant, Schopenhauer and Spenser.

Without laughter in our lives, we become too serious and inevitably we do not enjoy the pleasures that laughter can give us. As life is an expression of joy, we should laugh. We will then be in tune with nature as laughter comes from our heart. When you laugh, be it at life or at a funny story, you will feel a surge of happiness. Hence, let yourself laugh often. Laugh out loud. We should try to be like preschoolers as they laugh an estimated 450 times a day. Adults apparently laugh only 15 times a day. We should learn to let ourselves go.

BENEFITS OF LAUGHTER

"The person who knows how to laugh at himself will never cease to be amused."

Shirley McLaine

There are many advantages of laughing. While being safe and pleasurable, it promotes good health, both in body and spirit. It can lower blood pressure and improve the cardiovascular, respiratory and immune systems. When we laugh, our lung capacity expands and the blood circulates. Our oxygen consumption improves and our muscles relax. It is said that each time we laugh we tone 15 muscles. Laughter helps to activate the immune system and this in turn assists us to fight infection in a better way. It also stimulates digestion. Regular, hearty laughter helps lower heart disease. According to the *Daily Telegraph*, adult cancer patients exposed to funny situations have been shown to experience less pain, increased energy levels and improved mood.

Laughter helps to decrease stress and has been said to help relieve pain. It does so by helping the body produce endorphins. It can also help to dissipate anger and reduce irritation. When we laugh, we forget our problems and difficulties and we generally do not think of ill situations. Our attention is momentarily distracted and we become less tensed. We temporarily forget the pain, the fear, the tension and the seriousness of things. We feel hopeful about everything. Laughter definitely brightens our mood.

Laughter, in short makes us feel good. It can unlock energy flow. A good laugh can make us healthier and definitely happier. Laughter brings in powerful pleasure. It can put us at ease and make us more productive. Not only does laughter make us happier, it also helps us to be more creative.

31

IN DIFFICULT MOMENTS

"The sound of laughter is the vaulted dome of a temple of happiness."

Milan Kandera

When we laugh often, we tend to view life differently and change our attitude. In fact, it has been said that laughter makes us more pragmatic in our perceptions of the world. Laughter helps us to cope better during difficult times and it helps us to be more humble when we face success. It can help us survive grief and disappointment and get over anxiety and depression. When you are feeling low, you should try to smile and laugh. This will help to make your spirits feel better. We can view our problems differently and we will feel that we can control matters. Laughter can help us to face change in our lives and not to succumb to problems and difficulties. It will also guide us to live gracefully.

With laughter, difficult times become more controllable. Laughter between friends and acquaintances can help to develop goodwill and enhance friendships. It brings people together. Look on the bright side of life and try to see the funny side of things so you can laugh off the bad times. You will not be miserable if you can see the funny side of things. With a different perspective, we can actually turn a tragic situation into a funny one. Laughter is a skill we need to cultivate as we master the art of living. As Bill Cosby said, *"if you can laugh at it, you can survive it."*

PRACTICING LAUGHTER

Recognizing the benefits of laughter, Dr Madan Katria started laughter clubs. Today there are thousands of laughter clubs in India and in other countries. You can start a laughter club at your place of work or at home with your friends. Practice laughing at nothing at all. Just take a deep breath and laugh out loud. Tell funny stories to others. Learn to tell jokes and try and remember some good ones to share with your friends. However, please note that laughter is spontaneous and not just in response to jokes only. Laughter can be found in many human situations. Hence, you should make it a point to find one situation a day when you can have a hearty laugh. Learn to laugh more.

CULTIVATING LAUGHTER

We should try to laugh at ourselves. This has been described as a "liberating experience." If we can laugh at ourselves, we can in fact avoid being arrogant and pompous. Learn to laugh at the mistakes that you make which are funny. To help you appreciate and enhance your ability to laugh, it might help to assess your own laughter tendencies and the kind of humour that you prefer. Two important rules to observe as we practice laughter are that we should not laugh at the wrong times and that we should not, through our laughter, hurt the feelings of others.

To develop our ability to laugh we should view as much comedy as possible. Attend comedy shows, watch stand-up comedians or view them on television or at the cinema. Listening to people laugh can also be stimulating. Read comics and if you do this in the morning, for example by reading the comic strips in the newspapers, it will help you to feel happy. Take part in laughing contests.

"Laugh and the world laughs with you, weep and you weep alone."

E.W. Wilcox

Chapter 4

APPLY ZEAL

Zeal refers to enthusiastic devotion to a cause, ideal or goal and tireless diligence in its furtherance. It is a feeling of strong eagerness in favour of a cause. It comes from the Greek word, zelos which means ardent feeling. To be happy, we need to cultivate goals and causes enthusiastically and devotedly.

LIVE LIFE WITH A PURPOSE AND MEANING

We can attain happiness if we believe that our life has meaning and purpose. As a prisoner in a Nazi death camp, Viktor Frankl observed that people need a sense of purpose to maintain a will to live. To be happy, we need to recognize that our life has meaning and we need to believe that life itself has meaning. Bertrand Russell opinioned that people who view their life as a meaningful whole are happier than those who see it as a string of events with no particular theme or direction. Happiness comes if we live a life of purpose, loving and giving.

When your life has meaning, you find happiness. We will perceive ourselves and others differently if we have a significant meaning in our life. The way others view us will change. We therefore need to acquire a purpose in life. It has been said by some writers that an individual without a purpose or meaning in life will encounter problems. If we approach the work that we do with purpose and a sense of missionary zeal, we will feel happier and not regard work as a chore. Work would then be a part of us. The work that we perform, be it paid or otherwise, should be significant. It should be meaningful and important to us. When we feel that people need, appreciate and value our work, we feel happy.

COMMUNITY WORK

We should take a lesson from Mother Theresa who embarked on her cause of helping suffering people live or die with dignity one day after trying to get help for an ill woman in Kolkata. The hospitals that she took the poor woman to would not treat the woman and Mother Theresa took her back to her home and looked after her. She then dedicated her life to ease the pain of the suffering. When we help others and when we undertake community and voluntary services, we feel happy. Doing community work gives us a sense of purpose and makes us realize that we are part of a larger whole. Doing social work and undertaking acts of kindness will give an individual a meaningful and deep sense of happiness. The Dalai Lama stated that compassion for others is essential to happiness. Hence, when you help others you are, in fact helping yourself.

VOLUNTARY WORK

"You make a living by what you get, but you make a life by what you give."

Winston Churchill

Voluntary work gives a sense of purpose. You will feel good about yourself as you feel that your contributions are appreciated. When you volunteer, you will not feel bored and you will be happier than those people who do not volunteer. Hence, you should engage in volunteer activities. Do undertake voluntary work. When we help others and when we are good to other people, especially those who are less fortunate than us, we tend to feel happy. Volunteering also helps to relieve physical, emotional and mental tension. Make it a habit to do a good turn for someone every day. Brighten someone's day, if possible. You will feel happier when you do something for someone who needs cheering. You could send them a card; bring them soup, cookies, chocolates or flowers.

It is good to invest your time, energies and talents for a good cause. Cultivate a desire to help others, give real help and maintain a helpful attitude in all that you do. It is better, as they say, to give than to receive. You can give your time, money and skills to others. When you give to others you are, in fact, demonstrating love for others. You also generate joy, happiness and deep satisfaction. You will be rewarded by feeling fulfilled and you will develop a sense of purpose.

The selfless act of helping others is most gratifying. Giving therefore has been described as an active deed as it generates, creates and produces many good results. John Stuart Mills wrote in his autobiography, *"those only are happy...who have their minds fixed on some object other than their own happiness: on the happiness of others, on the improvement of mankind, even on some art or pursuit...Aiming thus at something else, they find happiness by the way."*

HELP OTHERS

To be happy, we need something to live for. Hence, be committed to a cause. Find a project with which you can be involved. Alternatively, set one up yourself and invite others to participate. If there is a community cause that you believe in strongly and for which you wish to serve, then you should use all your relevant strengths and virtues in work for this cause. Consider ways to increase the contributions that you make to this world. Be curious about life, the way it functions and operates. When you are interested in all this, you will be motivated to move, to be active and to initiate change.

If you sit and contemplate, brood and worry about yourself you will be unhappy. Instead, you should pick yourself up and join a programme where you can serve others. When you help someone to meet his or her need, you will experience happiness. We should try performing as many kind acts as possible in a day. Practice acts of kindness. Examples of acts of kindness would be:

- donating blood
- visiting an elderly person
- writing a thank you letter or
- preparing a gift for someone in need.

HAVE PASSION

> "A strong passion for any object will ensure success, for the desire of the end will point out the means."
>
> W. Hazlitt

We should also develop pursuits and activities which give us great passion. We need to develop passion in all that we do, in our work, hobbies, interests. Develop a passion for life. As you get excited about life, you should live, experience, see and do new things all the time. Our passion can inform and energize us. Happiness will come when we open up to the fullest for life, the gifts, possibilities and challenges which life can offer us. Let yourself be happy and engage in happy activities.

AVOID UNHAPPY EXPERIENCES

If you practice unhappy activities, then you will only continue to be unhappy. Do not focus on sad things. Do not regret past errors. Be strategic about this. Ask yourself what makes you happy and what makes you unhappy. Then work towards achieving the happy acts. Move from the unhappy experiences. Always reflect on the happy experiences which you, your family and friends have enjoyed in the past. This will help you to feel happy today. Be happy for what you have in life.

LIVE LIFE TO THE FULLEST

You should live everyday to the fullest. Don't tell yourself that "someday you will do this or do that". That day may never come. Live for today, live for the present. You do not want to wait till you are eighty to regret about all the things you have not done. Realize your dreams, make things happen. Change and move forward in life. **Feel happy, act happy and be happy today**. Do not wait for tomorrow or the next week. Tell yourself everyday that this is your last day on earth and you will live it well. When you do so, you will work to make it a great day, a special day, a fabulous day. Recognize that each day is important and you should enjoy every minute of the day. Every moment is precious and unique. The manner in which you spend your days is exactly the manner in which you spend your life.

Work on your tasks with passion and give every moment your best. Enjoy everything that you do, from the ordinary to the unusual. Make simple everyday chores seem special and most enjoyable. Identify what you are good at, your strengths and talents and use each one in a novel way. Teach yourself how to develop your optimism for life by learning to do away with thoughts which are negative.

DESIRE HAPPINESS

It has been said by others that when we establish a desire for something, we will work on acquiring it. Hence, we should make our happiness and the happiness of other people an important and fundamental desire for ourselves. To help us in this quest for happiness, we should value happiness. When we value happiness, we will then work towards achieving it. We will then be focused on achieving our greatest desire. Choose to be happy as this will help you continue to make choices to be happy. Making happy choices is important and relevant as we have many choices to make every day.

DEVELOP GOALS

"If you want to live a happy life tie it to a goal, not to people or things."

Albert Einstein

It helps if you wish to achieve happiness to develop meaningful goals for yourself. They should be desirable goals for every aspect of your life, for example, health, career, financial, attitude and relationships. These should be the aspects of your life which contribute to your happiness. Think of all the things you would like to do and work to realize them. The goals should be of significance to you. They should not conflict with each other. Make sure that the goals are specific and timely. If your goal is abstract it will be difficult to determine whether or not you have achieved the goal.

Once you have set your goals, you should devise a plan to achieve the goals, implement the plan and then check your progress. Once you see the progress that you are making, you will feel happy. A failure to achieve goals can cause you to feel frustrated and inadequate. This, in turn, will make you unhappy. To achieve our goals, we need to put in some work and we should aim to accomplish something each day.

VALUES AND BELIEFS

"Character is higher than intellect."

Ralph Waldo Emerson

Values and beliefs give us the motivation to pursue our daily activities. This is what fuels our passion and drive for life. Hence, to cultivate zeal in what we do, we need to practice and maintain beliefs and values. They will guide us and justify what we do. We can also use them as rules to live by. If we live our lives according to our values and beliefs we will attain happiness.

Values that are good to uphold include openness, cleanliness, orderliness, honesty, humility, courage, trust, freedom, harmony, security, persistence, generosity, health and variety. Cultivate and develop these values. Stand up for your values and beliefs.

Ask yourself what values and beliefs you currently have. Write these down on paper and then decide whether you would like to add some more in your life and whether you should develop others to greater levels. Maintain a record or journal to help you promote your values and beliefs.

AT WORK

"The true way to render ourselves happy is to love our work and find in it our pleasure."

Francoise de Motterville

Work with passion. Enjoy the work that you do. As you do so, try to help other people enjoy their work as well. Hence, you will need to approach people at work with friendliness. Interact with more people during your day. Cultivate friends at work. Work becomes enjoyable if you work with those you like. When

41

you work with others, try to understand their views, feelings and experiences. Ask others for their opinions, ideas, and suggestions. Compliment and praise others often as this will contribute to your overall happiness. Praise your colleagues and avoid putting others down.

When you see good qualities in other people, do not hesitate to show your appreciation. Let people know that they are producing good effective work. When you make someone feel good, you will also feel good. Send your friends and colleagues good wishes or a congratulatory message. Thank people in writing for something they may have done or may have given you. Send cards to friends and colleagues.

Avoid complaining. We should learn to be discreet, maintain integrity and keep private information confidential. Let others see through your actions that you keep all promises and that you are open to them. People will then trust, respect and admire you. It is wise not to engage in gossip. Instead, you should be open and honest. Do not look down on other people or engage in name-calling. All this will make you feel most unhappy.

TREAT OTHERS WELL

"The only way to have a friend is to be one."

Ralph Waldo Emerson

Respect other people's views, values and lifestyles as we are all different in the way we live our lives. Be passionate about developing trust bonds with your team members. Help others to develop themselves. Practice kindness and believe in people. The Buddhist monk, Matthieu Ricard concludes that we would be much happier if we would be nicer to each other. Encourage others to perform good work and to achieve their dreams. Avoid pettiness as it generates fault-finding in people and situations. If we are continually finding fault with others and if we allow pettiness to dominate the way we operate, we cannot then attain happiness. It is best to not practice pettiness and spitefulness as doing so will only make you feel unhappy. Pettiness will prevent you from achieving.

Give people the benefit of the doubt and do not assume the worst when you hear or see something bad about someone else. Neither should you feel paranoid that the people you are working with are just there to make things difficult to you or that they are always ready to find fault with you. This will only make your life at work very uncomfortable. Do not spread rumours and untruths as this can make you feel unhappy. The happy person avoids speaking ill of others. Generally, happy people smile at work very often and they enjoy themselves greatly. They are positive people who trust that if things are not going well, eventually the situation will improve. Treat people with dignity and support the dignity of others.

QUALITIES

> "For a person to build a rich and rewarding life for himself, there are certain qualities and bits of knowledge that he needs to acquire. There are also things, harmful attitudes, superstitions and emotions that he needs to chip away."
>
> Earl Nightingale

Other qualities which are good to use are patience, confidence, empathy, humour, creativity, optimism, energy, practicality, daring, honesty and generosity. In his book, *The Art of Happiness at Work*, the Dalai Lama says, *"be a good person, a kind person. Relate to others with warmth, human affection, with honesty and sincerity."* He regards kindness, caring and compassion as fundamental qualities.

Do not take credit for things you have not done. Instead, credit people for their good work. Confidence enables you to trust yourself to undertake challenges to take you to where you wish to go. It is essential to have confidence as it can help you succeed. Without confidence you could fail. Be curious too as this will propel you as you search for knowledge.

BELIEVE IN YOURSELF

As with the rest of your life, at work, practice responsibility for who you are, what you do and what happens. Face the challenges thrust upon you with zeal. Do not limit yourself at work. Banish any doubts or limitations that you may impose on yourself. Believe in yourself and your abilities. To be able to do something, you will first need to believe that you can do it. This will contribute to your happiness in your home life as well as work life. Use your abilities and talents to the fullest.

Give all of your attention to your tasks. Avoid thinking of other things that you should be doing as you work on the present task as this will only cause you to be unhappy. Take on new assignments and do not shy away from trying different things. This is the best way to keep energized at work. Your passion will fuel the energy to cope with all the new activities and new experiences.

DO YOUR BEST

Cultivate the passion to do your best at work and be proud of what you do. As Martin Luther King, Jr. said, "if you are called to be a street sweeper, sweep streets even as Michelangelo painted, or Beethoven composed music, or Shakespeare wrote poetry. Sweep streets so well that all the hosts of heaven and earth will pause to say, 'here lived a great sweeper who did his job well.'" Hence, you should be interested and concerned about what you are doing and you should perform well at your task. When we achieve and complete our tasks well, we generally feel better about ourselves. We feel relieved that the project, task or chore is completed and we are imbued with feelings of satisfaction and inner pride. When you attain success, you will feel confident about your abilities and you will feel that you are contributing to the organization.

YOUR WORK IS IMPORTANT

Be excited about your work. Passion and appreciation for your work will help you to develop a positive attitude to your work. Our mental attitude towards our work will determine whether we enjoy or dislike our work. To achieve happiness in our work, we need to like what we do. Develop a sense of purpose in what you do. Work in fact gives us a sense of purpose. Decide on what you like about the work that you do and the life that you have. If you feel that you are spending too much time on work, then put in more time on leisure. Be energetic and design an action plan to bring about change in your life or at your work place.

Tell yourself that you are going to make a difference at your workplace and throw yourself into your work with passion. Think of ways to contribute to your work. It is essential to remember that whatever your position is in the organization, what you do is important and will contribute to the success of the organization. If you can cooperate and work with others on a task, it is good to do so as it will help to make the task easier to accomplish and you will have fun working together.

PRESENTING YOUR IDEAS

When you present your ideas to others, be polite and smile. Plan how and what you are going to say ahead of time. This will help ensure that others will receive your ideas favourably. Present yourself in a happy way and be positive about your suggestions.

Make sure that you outline your ideas clearly and that you explain why your suggestions are good. In this way, you will feel happier about your work.

WORK SMART

Your job gives you the opportunity to demonstrate your talents and abilities, responsibility and productivity. Passion for your work will enable you to perform well. Do more than what is expected of you. Do more than the required. Work on your tasks with much effort and to the best of your ability. Have a variety of tasks. However, recognize that you do not have to do everything on your own. Acquire the skills of delegation. If you undertake everything on your own, you will soon feel stressed, overburdened and in no time, you will suffer from burn-out. When this happens, you cannot feel happy. Your job will give you the opportunity to demonstrate your talents and abilities, your sense of responsibility and your productivity.

Strike out and go the extra mile. You alone have the power to inspire yourself, so do your work with passion.

Chapter 5

HAVE ZEST

"Three Grand Essentials to Happiness in this Life are Something to Do, Something to Love and Something to Hope for."

Joseph Addison

DEFINITION OF ZEST

Zest has been defined as spirited enjoyment; gusto; feeling of pleasure and enthusiasm. It has also been defined as the quality of being exciting, enjoyable and interesting. We experience pleasure from different sources. For example, we experience pleasure from being with our friends, from aesthetic beauty, from art, from consuming food and drink. We also get pleasure from exercising and participating in physical activity and from any achievement we may make. We can engage ourselves in situations which are exciting, enjoyable and interesting. All this will make us feel happy and give us an enjoyable life.

CULTIVATE HAPPY ATTITUDES

To have zest for life, for living and for being, we need to cultivate attitudes that give us pleasure and enthusiasm. We need to use our mind and our intelligence to generate these attitudes which will help us to achieve happiness. Our attitudes influence our emotional responses as well. Our thoughts decide on the kind of emotions that we display. When we think of unhappy thoughts, we will be unhappy. If we think of happy, pleasant thoughts, we will be happier. We should therefore learn to dismiss unpleasant thoughts and replace them with happy, pleasant thoughts. Challenge your negative thoughts and analyse whether you need to be negative.

The real source of happiness lies in our minds and not in external circumstances. As has been said by others, how we view the world is how it will be. Our attitude will direct the way we live and influence our achievements. Cultivate an upbeat attitude and apply this in all that you undertake. This is guaranteed to bring you great success. As someone once said, the presence, absence and depth of happiness is determined by our internal attitudes. Unhappy people dwell on unpleasant happenings which they have experienced. These experiences are locked in our subconscious mind and they affect the way we face life. We should not allow these unhappy, unpleasant experiences restrict us from reaching out and being happy. To enjoy our life fully, we should concentrate on what is doing well and what is working rather than to give our attention to what is not working and not performing well.

AVOID NEGATIVE THOUGHTS AND PREJUDICES

"Prejudices, it is well known, are most difficult to eradicate from the heart whose soil has never been loosened or fertilized by education; they grow there, firm as weeds among rocks."

Charlotte Bronte

Happiness is an attitude that can be generated within oneself. Happy people are optimistic and outgoing. To be optimistic, learn to recognize and get rid of all thoughts which are devastating

48

and bad. Happy people will, instead, search for knowledge that will keep them happy. Avoid negative, cynical thinking. When you are less critical, you will experience peace of mind. It has been said by others before that if you change your thinking, your situation and life will change. Do not accept prejudices and stereotypes as they cripple your thinking. This will also prevent you from enjoying experiences that help you to be a happier person. Banish unpleasant thoughts and think pleasant ones instead. This will make you feel happier and be better.

DECIDE TO BE HAPPY

"Today is life — the only life you are sure of. Make the most of today. Get interested in something. Shake yourself awake. Develop a hobby. Let the winds of enthusiasm sweep through you. Live today with gusto."

Dale Carnegie

You are responsible for your happiness and for the way in which you interact with others and cope with situations. You can choose to be happy or sad. It is a choice that you make for yourself. Decide to be happy and this in itself will help to generate happiness for you. When we wake up in the morning we should tell ourselves that "Today is going to be a great day, a perfect day." Then we should work on making it a great day. Think of happy thoughts first thing in the morning and tell yourself that you will have a happy day filled with many happy moments.

Start the day on a positive note and this will help you to feel happy all day. It helps to read inspirational quotes and stories in the morning. Your thoughts are very important as they influence the quality of your life. So be selective and only think of happy, positive issues. Think of happy things, situations, and events all the time. If something miserable comes to mind, throw it out. Do not dwell on it. Do not think about ill matters or aches and pains as this will make you feel depressed. Think of happiness itself as this should make you feel happy.

Commit to memory that you should feel very happy every day. This would help you make happiness a habit! Tell yourself that you are happier than what you actually feel. During the day, just repeat a statement like this one, "I am very happy." As we repeat this, we will accept the idea and we will start to feel happier. Other statements that you could say to yourself and which will help you to feel happy are, "I feel wonderful" and "I feel good." Express these sentiments in as many different ways as possible.

"He is happy that knoweth not himself to be otherwise."

Thomas Fuller

WE ARE RESPONSIBLE FOR OUR CHOICES

We need to recognize that we are responsible for our own responses to events, situations, people and places. If we see things in an irrational manner, then even if it is not such a difficult or intense problem, we will experience a great deal of anxiety and even some pain. Generally, it is our interpretation of the problem, rather than the problem itself, which causes us to be unhappy. Accept whatever happens as this will give you more control over changing things. We should view life as opportunity and that challenges which come before us are not overly difficult but are merely there to test us.

We should recognize that we are responsible for our choices. We make decisions which can cause us happiness or pain. Hence, we cannot blame others for our unhappiness. As such, we are responsible for our own happiness. Take control of your life. Make positive choices and change your life. Change the way you respond to the challenges which come your way. Look for the happy and beautiful aspects in every situation you encounter.

BE POSITIVE

"There is little difference in people, but that little difference makes a big difference. That little difference is attitude. The big difference is whether it is positive or negative."

Mark Twain

One can achieve success if one has a positive attitude, thinks positively and is not overcome by challenges and difficulties. Not only should we think positively, we should also have positive expectations and undertake positive actions. Only then can we enjoy good outcomes and happy results. When you experience something positive, enjoy it and accept it. You are responsible for your happiness and the way in which you interact with others and cope with situations.

OPTIMISM

*"Optimism is the faith that leads to achievement.
Nothing can be done without hope and confidence."*

Helen Keller

To have enthusiasm in what we do, we need to focus on the positive. Ignore the negative and habitually develop an optimistic attitude. Learn to get rid of worries and concerns. A positive state of mind is essential. Happiness depends on what we think. As Abraham Lincoln said, ***"most people are about as happy as they make up their minds to be."*** Think about happiness, talk about it with other people and behave as if you expect to be happy. Tell yourself that from henceforth you will be happy.

Being optimistic and having an open mind helps us to develop happiness as we can look at our problems more positively. We will not allow our problems to make us feel anxious and subsequently be unhappy. We can make our life good or we can make it bad. As the popular statement states, we can look at a glass half-filled with water and see it as half empty or half full. To be happy, you need the ability and skills to be optimistic. Martin Seligman has conducted research on optimism and his findings indicate that optimism can help people pass examinations, stay longer in a job and keep and look healthier after forty-five. So you should hope for the best always and life will be good.

LOOK FOR THE RAINBOW

A positive attitude will make us stronger people. This makes us live through difficult periods. We will be better able to cope with failures and mistakes. With every experience which we encounter, we will look for something good. Practice what is commonly expected of us that after a storm, look for the rainbow. We will take each day as it comes along, live it and enjoy ourselves. Each day is a new day which will bring us joy and we should appreciate this and relish each little aspect of the joy we experience. Our lives will be transformed and we will be truly happy. According to Norman Vincent Peale, **"the person who sends out positive thoughts activates the world around him positively and draws back to himself positive results."**

YOUR ATTITUDE MAKES A DIFFERENCE

"Happiness is an attitude. We either make ourselves miserable, or happy and strong. The amount of work is the same."

Francesca Reigler

A positive attitude toward life and others is definitely a requirement for a life of happiness. Being positive will definitely help us to be happy. When we fill ourselves with negativity, we will not be able to acquire great levels of happiness. Teach yourself to avoid all negative thoughts. When a negative thought comes to you, think of it as being put to you by someone who is intent on making you feel unhappy. Then fight the thought and do not let it take centre stage.

In their personal and professional life, happy people exhibit a great deal of assurance and confidence. People who are positive can see opportunities in many situations. Hence, they do better. Your attitude makes a big difference in your life. Being positive is something we need to develop over time.

POSITIVE PEOPLE ATTRACT OTHERS

We do not need to have a perfect life in order to be happy. Be satisfied for the way you are choosing to live your life. We need to cultivate a positive concept of our self-worth and a positive vision of everything around us, the world and the events in our life. Be the optimistic, positive person at home, in your place of work and in your social group. Happy people are also drawn to other happy people. People are encouraged by your positive nature and they will enjoy being with you.

According to Thomas Blakeslee, "good attitudes affect happiness and bring pleasure and wellbeing, which are vital for good health. Attitudes affect your appearance as well as your health. Smile lines look a lot better than frown lines."

HANDLING PROBLEMS

To develop a positive outlook, we should maintain a sense of humour and put fun into everything that we do. When we approach our problems and challenges, we should remind ourselves of our purpose and mission. It is useful to remind ourselves when faced with problems that we are not the only one experiencing difficulties in this world. Everyone experiences problems, disappointments and pain from time to time. Today's problem is just one small hiccup. Always look on the bright side of things.

We should also tell ourselves that we have the choice to be negative or positive. We should cultivate confidence to deal with the frustrations, sadness and disappointments that may come our way. The best decision that we can make for ourselves is to remove and banish all negative thoughts and emotions. Only then can we be optimistic, positive and courageous. Once we are calm and serene we can face life's challenges. When you daydream, focus on happy dreams. You will not only think happy but be happy as well.

Feeling good is important and essential to happiness. If we look at life and expect the best from it, we will be much happier than if we looked at life expecting that things will be bad. Worrying will not help us to feel happy. Neither will it help us to solve problems or correct situations which are not good. Instead of worrying over something, just take action to solve or correct it.

EMOTIONS TO AVOID

"Feelings are much like waves, we can't stop them from coming but we can choose which one to surf."

Jonaton Martensson

Avoid being angry every day. You can never be happy if you get angry easily. Avoid harbouring feelings of hate in your heart. Other feelings that we should avoid experiencing are superiority, egoism and pretension. We should avoid putting others down, bullying, sneering and being violent. Try to minimize the unpleasant emotions of fear, sadness and disgust. Be in control of your emotions and enjoy a balanced life. This will bring you happiness. Try to be more conscious of your own emotions and how they affect you and others around you. To do so, you will need to recognize how the different moods surface, the physical symptoms that come with each mood and the way in which you can change your mood.

BANISH CERTAIN FEELINGS

"For a person to build a rich and rewarding life for himself, there are certain qualities and bits of knowledge that he needs to acquire. There are also things, harmful attitudes, superstitions, and emotions that he needs to chip away."

Earl Nightingale

We should also try to banish feelings which do not help us to develop happiness. These include the following: guilt, shame, anxiety, contempt, doubt, jealousy, self-pity, hate, disgust, stress, depression and envy. These destructive states of mind should not be entertained and you should cultivate peaceful ones. When we are unhappy because of the negative feelings that we maintain within ourselves, we become distrustful of others, we become inward-looking and also defensive about ourselves.

LIFE BEGINS NOW

Live in the present and recognize that life begins right now, at this very moment, at this time. One exercise that you can undertake is to sit and focus on feeling happy. Just repeat to yourself, "I feel happy" and think of happy, pleasant thoughts. Set aside some time for practice happiness sessions when you can think happy thoughts and select great, happy thoughts.

BE GRATEFUL

"Happiness is the spiritual experience of living every minute with love, grace and gratitude."

Dennis Waitley

Develop a sense of gratitude as it will help you to be happy. If we are grateful for what we have, for the life that we lead, for the friends that we have and for the possessions we have acquired, we will acquire more in life and we will also meet other good people. Avoid feeling envious of others. When you do so, you believe that other people are better than you. You then become dissatisfied with everything in your life. This will make you feel unhappy. Avoid looking at other people's lifestyle and evaluating your success by this. Focus on what you currently have and enjoy every part of it. Be grateful even for small and simple things. Each night you could record three things that went well and review why they went well.

Be grateful and thankful for your life throughout the day. Be grateful not just for the things which happen to you but also for the things which do not happen to you. There is no need to compare what you have in life with what other people may have. If you appreciate what you have over what you do not have you will enjoy much happiness. Happy people are grateful for many different things. If you appreciate all the good things in your life, you will definitely feel happy. Happy people understand what it means to be grateful. Even when they are experiencing problems, they can still find something for which to be grateful. For example, they may appreciate just being alive. We all have things in our lives for which we are grateful. In fact, there is much for which we can be thankful.

Happy people are grateful people. They find life enjoyable and exciting. They are enthusiastic about everything that they undertake and experience. With gratitude, we develop open minds and we are more able to work with others and help them and we are inspired to find creative solutions to problems. Make friends with people who are grateful and who motivate, inspire and encourage others.

MUCH TO BE GRATEFUL FOR

"Let us rise and be thankful, for if we didn't learn a lot today, at least we learned a little, and if we didn't learn a little, at least we didn't get sick, and if we got sick, at least we didn't die; so let us all be thankful."

Buddha

First, we should be grateful for being alive, for being able to think, to do, and to be. We are fortunate to be able to read, to write and to speak for there are many who are visually handicapped, who are not able to speak and whose hearing is impaired. We should also be happy that we have modern amenities in life when there are many who live in squalor and poverty. For those of us who enjoy peace and security, we should be grateful when we see so many others who live in war-torn countries. We should also be grateful for the roof over our heads when there are so many people in this world who have no homes and live on the streets.

A good exercise to use is to decide on some things for which you are grateful. This could be very ordinary items or features, like your eyes, your family or your pet dog. It should include things that we often take for granted. At an appointed time each day, you could think about these pleasures that you have and this will help to make you feel happier. When faced with so much to be grateful about, it is difficult to feel miserable and depressed. It is definitely not possible to be grateful and unhappy.

GRATITUDE EXERCISES

"Gratitude helps you to grow and expand; gratitude brings joy and laughter into your life and into the lives of those around you."

Eileen Caddy

Maintain a gratitude journal. Each day you should think of five things that you are grateful for in your life. This will compel you each day to consider some positive aspect of your life, be it your health, friends, family, education and conditions around you. In turn, you will enjoy a greater sense of well-being.

Another exercise that you can undertake is to spend an hour writing down everything for which you are grateful. You may encounter difficulties at having to write for an hour. Every day after this, add at least one other item to the list that you have prepared. You could, if you like, prioritize the items on your list. This exercise will help you to be happier.

To help you to be happy write a thank you letter to someone who has been good to you. Visit someone who has also assisted you in some way and who you have not thanked properly. When you acknowledge the assistance and contributions of others, you will feel happy. Recognize that you can be happy with what you have. Be content with your life and accept your circumstances. Little can be achieved by thinking all the time of the people and issues that upset you. It will make you feel unhappy and less satisfied with your life.

AVOID MOANING AND GROANING

If you complain all the time, you will soon be very unhappy. You will not be able to institute change and improve your lot.

Moaning, groaning and complaining are negative emotions which prevent you from being objective about life. Instead they make you feel discouraged and depressed. You will only feel unhappy with yourself, what you do and the life you lead. People who moan and groan are often very powerful in that they can influence others to be miserable.

When you hear yourself moaning, groaning or complaining, stop yourself immediately. If you are in the habit of complaining all the time, give up the habit. Avoid blaming, finger-pointing and accusing, all of which are evidence of poor attitudes and unproductive behaviour. Do not allow yourself to be overcome with anger and resentment. Keep hate well away from you. Your health will deteriorate if you maintain ill feelings and are hostile all the time.

BE GRACIOUS

"If a man be gracious or courteous to strangers, it shows he is a citizen of the world, and that his heart is no island cut off from other lands, but a continent that joins to them."

Francis Bacon

Avoid constantly criticizing others. Try to be gracious at all times and do not take away their dignity from them. Learn to forgive others because if you are unforgiving, you will be unhappy and bitter. You will also resent others. Forget the issue once you have forgiven someone. It does not pay to be consumed with self-pity and to constantly worry. Do not worry if things are not fair. Just get on with your life and take action. Neither should you be afraid of people, places, the future and life itself. Blaming other people for what happens to you will not help you. There is no point in thinking that the whole world is against you.

FOCUS ON KINDNESS

"Constant kindness can accomplish much. As the sun makes ice melt, kindness causes misunderstanding, mistrust, and hostility to evaporate."

Albert Schweitzer

We should direct our attention to the good in life. Focus on kindness and appreciation. Regularly, perform acts of kindness for others. Think of other people and reach out to those in need. When we help other people to be happier, we will in turn increase our own happiness. Be conscious all the time for ways to show kindness and help other people. Holding a door open for someone behind you is a small act of kindness. But an act like this one would make you feel satisfied with yourself and also make the other person feel good. When we are happy with ourselves, we tend to help others as well. It has also been proven that when we do good deeds, we also feel good. Be kind to others and you will experience a sense of fulfillment.

COMPLIMENT OTHERS

"A compliment is verbal sunshine."

Robert Orben

Compliment people as this will make you feel happy. Make it a habit to give a compliment at least once a day. Tell or write to your friends cards highlighting something about them that you consider excellent and that you appreciate very much. Expressing our compliments about someone else's good qualities is a more productive and happy exercise than merely looking at things which are annoying. Say to people you care about, "I love you." It will make both you and them feel happy.

60

Be happy for others and enjoy their happiness. You will then be filled with much joy and happiness. Be thoughtful and help others, especially those who cannot help you. Be generous and help others to realize their potential. We should try to avoid petty arguments and any energy draining deliberations that are not about significant issues. These things are unproductive and toxic.

TOXIC PERSONALITIES

"No person is your friend who demands your silence, or denies your right to grow."

Alice Walker

Stay away from toxic people, that is, people who are negative and energy-draining. Toxic personalities do nothing but make you feel bad about yourself and about life in general. These are the people who will make you feel tired and lacking in energy. Toxic personalities will only make you respond negatively which will make it difficult for you to feel happy. You should instead mix with people who are happy, vibrant and have common interests with you as they will make you happy. Be with people you can trust and whom you believe are not selfish and have goodwill towards you.

PRACTICE FORGIVENESS

"Forgiveness
Is the mightiest sword
Forgiveness of those you fear
Is the highest reward
When they bruise you with words
When they make you feel small
When it's hardest to take
You must do nothing at all."

Jane Eyre

61

Learn to forgive yourself and others. Accept yourself. Focus and develop all that is good in you. Review what other people like about you and consider good about you. Work on these aspects and you'll be happy. Forgive your friends' short-comings. It is important to like yourself and others as this makes you feel happy. You need to respect yourself and what you do.

It is good to try to relate to your feelings, needs, and desires. Only then will you be able to relate to other people. Avoid judging other people and behaving in a judgemental way as this will make you unhappy. Try to see the best in others. Try to relate effectively to others. Cultivate good and stable rela-tionships and try to care for other people.

MAINTAINING FRIENDSHIPS

"A friend is one who knows us, but loves us anyway."

Jerome Cumming

Cultivate friends who are different from and more interesting than you. You will be able to learn much from them and in turn, you will become a much more interesting person. Make it a point to meet people and make friends everywhere you go. Developing a friendship is not an easy, simple task. It requires effort, hard work, care, time and dedication to develop a friendship. When you have friends, make sure you nurture your closest friend-ships. This may not be easy for many people. Here are some suggestions as to what you can do when you wish to develop friendships.

- Avoid making judgments of other people, being critical, envi-ous or competing with others.
- Avoid feeling jealous, resentful or being angry. Try not to feel resentful of people.

- Do not accept slights and insults.
- Give love, be nice to others.
- Learn from others and do not hesitate to assist people.
- Learn to give to others and to forgive others as well.
- Try to understand your friends.
- When and if you need to make an apology to anyone, do so gracefully and with dignity.
- Be generous and kind with people.
- Learn to live a rich life filled with grace and goodwill.
- Give your friends hugs often.
- Do not take those closest to you for granted.
- Respect everyone with whom you interact.
- Try to care about others and find joy in their joy.

REACHING OUT TO OTHERS

"Every friend represents a world in us, a world possibly not born until they arrive, and it is only by this meeting that a new world is born."

Anais Nin

You should value the time that you spend with other people and if they need cheering up, do not hesitate to help them cheer up. Reach out to people at all times. Look for friendly faces wherever you are as this will make you feel safe and comfortable. When a person leaves you, let the person feel good and be better off for having been with you. It is also good to make others feel important. This means that you should be good, kind and loving to others at all times. To be so, it helps to always expect and find the best in people.

Be polite at all times. Never be rude, boring, selfish or tiresome. Greet everyone you meet, your colleagues, neighbours and others with a cheery hello. Return all phone calls and answer all e-mail messages. Let those with whom you work know when you observe and appreciate their talents and abilities. When they are with you and talking to you, remember to look them in the eye. Have one good conversation with someone each day. Always think and ask after others.

CONFIDING IN OTHERS

Being close to people ensures that you can share your thoughts and feelings with them. Be open with your friends and do not stay away from people. Confiding is good for you. When you confide in someone, you will know that you will be understood. From time to time let your friends know that you will play together and share together.

THINGS TO DO

"Blessed are those who have the gift of making friends, for it is one of God's best gifts. It involves many things, but above all, the power of going out of one's self, and appreciating whatever is noble and loving in another."

Thomas Hughes

Here is a list of things which you can do to develop good relationships with your friends.

- Cultivate friendships and meet with your friends from time to time.
- Invite your friends to a party that is not just well organized but spectacular and fun-filled, one that people will remember for always.
- Organize a thank-you party for your friends. Tell them how much you enjoy their company.
- Write to people who have helped you or been nice to you and thank them for their kindness and support. If you have good thoughts for others, make them known.

- Have a long conversation with a friend, a spouse or a partner at least once a week. Be open with each other about your feelings about things and in this way, you can handle many of the experiences that you may, encounter in your life.
- To feel happy, we need to share the happenings in our life with others. Talking through your problems with a friend or just catching up with each other will make you feel good. Having close supportive relationships will help you to feel happy. Happy people understand that such relationships are valuable and relevant to our sense of happiness.
- Call a friend you have not seen or heard from for sometime. The people you have known for a long time are very often your best friends. Friends you have known from the past and with whom you associate great memories will give you a rich significant experience.
- Support your friends by giving help and comforting them when they need assistance. You will feel good doing this. People feel happy and great about themselves if they feel close to other people. Our sense of happiness is increased when we have many good friends, many close friends and when our relationships with our family members and with colleagues and neighbours are good.
- We all have a deep desire to feel needed. Hence, consider those who depend on you for your friendship, care and help. It helps sometimes to generate a list of all the people you have good relations with and for whom you care. You make a difference to the lives of others.
- Establish new friendships. Choose friends who will make you feel good. Enjoy and even relish the attention that they give you. You will receive and enjoy many rewards from this. For example, you will find yourself energized, happy and challenged. Ideally your friends should be positive, happy people who love life.

GOOD FRIENDS

"Friends are helpful not only because they will listen to us, but because they will laugh at us. Through them we learn a little objectively, a little modesty, a little courtesy. We learn the rules of life and become better players of the game."

Will Durant

Good friends can make you feel fabulous. They add value to your life and make you feel happy. They make life worth living. Recognize that there will always be differences between people. If we are flexible, we will be able to adapt and accept these differences.

Our manners toward others should always be pleasant. Greet people cheerfully and always wish them well. Remember to wish them to have a good day. When you are with someone make sure that you give them your full attention. Listen carefully to what they have to say. Hug your friends and family members as hugs help to express your love for them. We need hugs ourselves as they help us grow emotionally. When you provide a reason for others to be happy, you too will be happier.

BE WITH PEOPLE WHO LOVE YOU

"One word frees us of all the weight and pain of life: the word is love."

Sophocles

Be with people who will give you love and make you feel good. Give the people who make you feel good top priority in your life. The good relationships that we cultivate with others will give us much joy and comfort, a good sense of security and love. They will help us to get through difficult periods. Supportive social connections are fundamental to feeling good. Friendships

66

affect our sense of well being. People with close caring families and friends and who belong to some kind of community tend to be happier and more satisfied with life.

Friendships become more important to us as we get older. Over time, we lose our friends because we may decide that we do not need each other, because of different interests, of distance and perhaps because we have not made the effort to keep in touch and build upon our friendship. Attend or organize class reunions to be with your friends. The pleasure you get from being with each other will stimulate you and make you feel happy. Remember that it is the people who love you who will bring you much happiness. As **Victor Hugo said,** *"the greatest happiness of life is the conviction that we are loved — loved for ourselves, or rather loved in spite of ourselves."*

COMMUNICATING WITH OTHERS

"To effectively communicate, we must realize that we are all different in the way we perceive the world and use this under-standing as a guide to our communication with others."

Anthony Robbins

Do not be aggressive with your friends and family. When discussing an issue with others, remind yourself that the issue is not as important as the people with whom you are discussing the issue. Consider the tone of voice that you adopt and the words that you use as they speak volumes. Be aware of your body language as well. They may be small things but their impact is great. When engaged in discussions, make sure that you ask questions and that you consider the answers that you get appropriately.

Do not be too hasty to disagree with the answers that you receive. Avoid dominating the discussion or conversation. Try to be agreeable so that others will find it easier to interact with you. When someone makes a critical comment or an angry remark, do not answer immediately. Pause before you make a response. A good guide is to count up to ten before you answer the person. Control your anger and any tendency that may be disruptive.

BE MODEST

It helps in relationships if we cultivate a modest attitude. When we are modest, people will reach out to us and wish to help us. No one likes being with arrogant people. We should also avoid boasting as people do not like being near those who boast. People who boast are generally insecure and feel inferior. They try to make up for this by boasting. Be sincere in your thoughts and actions. When you communicate with others, always be honest as this will save you much anxiety later. When we tell lies, we tend to be unhappy. Be a good sport with everyone. Be thoughtful and polite with others. Do not hesitate to ask for forgiveness when you need to do so. You will experience a good feeling, a sense of calm and peace.

BE WITH OTHERS

As human beings we need to belong to groups, to others. We have a psychological need to be part of a bigger unit. When you are a member of a group, you learn to cultivate good relationships with others. This will help you interact well with others, feel less lonely and more secure. Discuss your problems with others as, by doing so, you can obtain a different perspective and you will find solutions to your problem. We can definitely learn from other people. As social beings, we need to discuss our problems with each other. It is important too to be able to share your desires, aspirations and feelings with your family and friends. The support and understanding that we receive from them will make us feel happier with ourselves. If we do not share with others, we will feel lonely and misunderstood. This makes us unhappy.

When we communicate with others, we should practice good listening habits. This will help us to avoid any misunderstanding and in this way we will feel happier. Do not hesitate to ask the other person to repeat something if you do not understand what the person is saying. If you can share your concerns and needs openly you should enjoy a happier relationship.

FAMILY RELATIONSHIPS

"Families are the cornerstone of our society. They surround us with love and acceptance, and gird us with enduring support and strength. They give us a sense of purpose and fulfillment in life. No amount of wealth or material success can substitute for a happy family. We must, therefore, nurture the ties of kinship everyday, and not just during festival occasions..."

Lee Hsien Loong, Prime Minister of Singapore

Family relationships contribute much to the happiness that we enjoy in life. It is therefore essential to maintain close contacts with your family and to keep them informed of what is happening in your life. Organise and value all the special occasions that you have with your family members. Take photographs at these special occasions and keep a record of them. Talk to each other of those memorable occasions.

RELATIONSHIP WITH YOUR SPOUSE

"Only choose in marriage a woman whom you would choose as a friend if she were a man."

Joseph Joubert

69

To enjoy a good relationship with your spouse you need to work on that relationship. Here are some suggestions:

- Be a friend to your spouse.
- Be kind to your spouse.
- Hold hands with each other as touch is good for the emotions.
- Implement, develop and enhance the following factors that contribute towards happiness in a marriage: love, laughter, communication, mutual respect, fun and pleasure at being together.
- Share your feelings with each other openly.
- Be honest with each other.
- Listen to each other.
- Be romantic towards each other.
- Write a letter or a card expressing your love.
- Organise a special dinner or outing for the two of you.
- Learn to work with each other.
- Support and respect each other as best as can be.
- Unwind before you reach home everyday. In this way, you will be able to concentrate attentively to what happens at home, to what anyone may say to you and to what tasks you may have to undertake. This will contribute towards your happiness.
- Organize your life such that you can spend adequate time with your family.
- Develop a healthy work-life relationship and this will contribute to your overall happiness.

RELATIONSHIP WITH CHILDREN

"The soul is healed by being with children."

Frodor Dostoevsky

When and if you do have children, cherish and love them. Demonstrate this to them physically by giving them hugs and kisses. Write little notes to motivate and tell how much you love them. Put notes in their school bags to tell how much you appreciate them. Compliment your child as this will help your child feel valuable and important. Compliments make people feel happy and good about themselves. Always make children feel secure. Enhance their self esteem at all times. Children need discipline and morals and it is therefore important to provide this.

Develop rules for them and set high moral standards. Communicate with your children often and do not avoid discussing moral issues with them. Guide them to be responsible global citizens. Make it a point to have meals with them during the week. As you eat, you can talk to them and they will learn how to communicate and discuss issues. This is also a very good way to generate informal learning and such activities help to strengthen family ties. If you have children who are balanced, happy and loving, you have achieved much indeed in life.

CARING FOR OTHERS

We also need to care about other people and to be cared for by others as well. Tell your friends how important they are to you. Tell them how much you care for them. With mutual appreciation, you can foster good relationships. Encourage your friends and acquaintances. Try to avoid developing relationship problems.

"Do not be afraid of showing your affection.
Be warm and tender, thoughtful and affectionate.
Men are more helped by sympathy, than by
service; love is more than money, and a kind word
will give more pleasure than a present."

Sir John Lubbock

RELATIONSHIP PROBLEMS

Do not hate others. When we do so, we only bring that person close to us and this is something we wish to avoid. The best thing to do is to eliminate the person from our thoughts. Bad relationships can cause you to be unhappy. When you get upset with someone and might be very angry with the person for the mistake that he or she may have made, avoid getting too worked up over this. Do not scold the person relentlessly as this generates resentment on yourself, establishes a lack of cohesion within the office, family, social group or community team and it destroys enthusiasm. You end up feeling stressed and unhappy.

Avoid negative emotions like fear, disgust, repulsion and hatred. They erode any sense of happiness that you may be experiencing. Do not use force on others in order to obtain things. This will make you feel exhausted and eventually you become unhappy.

BE EXTROVERTED

To have zest in life and to react more positively to situations, it helps if we are extroverted in personality. Extroverts associate with people more easily, interact and engage in social activities more often and they tend to be happier people. They are more positive and are generally more satisfied with their situations. Avoid being isolated and lonely as this can make you feel even more unhappy. Try to be with other people often. To be happy we need to love and be loved and we need to establish connections with others. Fill your life with love.

CULTIVATE HIGH SELF-ESTEEM

"Nothing profits more on self-esteem, grounded on what is just and right."

John Milton

To be more outgoing in personality and to have a wider social network, we should also have high self-esteem. To be truly happy, we need to like ourselves, have self-respect and accept ourselves for whom and what we are as people. When you can love and accept yourself the way you are, you can then love and accept anyone else the way they are. We should accept our looks, intelligence, emotions and actions. Stop criticizing yourself and trying to get yourself to achieve the more difficult tasks. Be kind and patient with yourself. Connect with yourself and look after your mental, spiritual and emotional health. Do not be a perfectionist either. Make friends with yourself. In fact, we should love ourselves and be happy with ourselves. If you treat yourself well, everyone else will also treat you well. Having high self-esteem and feeling good about oneself will contribute to lasting happiness.

To enjoy high self esteem, we should look at what we are good at and appreciate ourselves. For example, draw up a list of all your good qualities. Appreciating what we have makes us satisfied internally. We should tell ourselves that we are unique and that we really count and matter. Consider the good qualities that you have and congratulate yourself for this. From time to time remind yourself of your achievements in life. It pays to know your self-worth. Avoid having unrealistic expectations of yourself.

If you like yourself it will be easier to engage in social interactions. In fact, you will enjoy participating in social exchanges. With this comes, enthusiasm, pleasure and zest. When you are happy with yourself and love yourself more, others around you will respond with love and happiness for you too. High self esteem does lead to greater happiness. It has been said that low self-esteem contributes to depression. People with low self-esteem tend to brood, be depressed, be antagonistic and are withdrawn. Learn to like yourself and others.

CULTIVATE PEACE OF MIND

*"In the final analysis, the hope of every person
is simply peace of mind."*

The Dalai Lama

To achieve a positive attitude, to be more relaxed, to have higher self-esteem, be less stressed, be more optimistic, friendly and confident, we need to have peace of mind. With peace of mind, our relationships with others will also improve. When we have peace of mind and when we feel good about our-selves, we will be able to perform well at our work and we will want to do well at it. We will also make good bosses and work well with others.

When we worry about what others think of us and that whatever we do is never ever good enough for others, we will be unhappy. We should not allow other people's opinion of us affect us. Be confident as confident people are happy people. Always tell yourself that you can achieve. When you are successful, you will feel good about yourself and also feel happy.

KEEP LEARNING

*"The purpose of learning is growth, and our minds, unlike our
bodies, can continue growing as long as we live."*

Mortimer Adler

To enjoy life and to find things interesting, we need to develop ourselves morally, intellectually and emotionally. We need to acquire knowledge and wisdom. Research on happiness suggests that we can find happiness from developing new skills. Learning something new and acquiring a skill we could not do previously is motivational, interesting and enjoyable. Hence, it is necessary that we embark on learning new skills and attending courses.

We can also acquire knowledge and improve our personal development by learning new ideas, learning from the media, keeping up with events on the news and through reading and surfing the internet. The more knowledge and skills that we acquire, the more capable and confident we become as people. This, in turn, will make us happier with ourselves. To find enduring happiness, we need to be on the constant look-out for opportunities to develop our skills. We can then use our new skills to perform better and faster at our job or extend and develop the tasks associated with it.

Knowing alone is not enough. We need to do things differently. We should also look for new challenges that are suitable for us. As we meet new challenges we grow, become more confident and happier. Learn to use a computer so that you can enjoy the challenge of using technology and learn how to acquire information and interact globally. Use technology to enhance your life. Do not let it dominate you. Learn a new language and make it a habit to spend a small amount of time each day learning the language. Learn to play a musical instrument as this will challenge you as you enjoy the music that you can generate.

Be prepared to continually learn new skills and acquire new knowledge. Learning new things contributes to our happiness. Make it a habit to learn something new everyday. As you learn, your mind keeps active and alert. When you cultivate the habit of learning something new everyday, you will be happy and will approach each day with vigour.

SKILLS OF LEARNING

> "The illiterate of the twenty-first century will not be those who cannot read and write, but those who cannot learn, unlearn and relearn."

> Alvin Toffler

Acquire the skills of learning. With an "I can do it" attitude, you will be able to learn much and enjoy many happy experiences. Be aware of ways to adapt, acquire and implement new knowledge. Learn how to probe for information, look for it and retain it. Give yourself plenty of opportunity to enjoy hands-on experiences. Expose yourself to intellectual stimulation through various media. Read, listen and learn as much as possible.

Stimulate your thinking, curiousity, creativity and aesthetic appreciation by watching television programmes and reviewing computer programmes on news, documentaries, exploration, travel, arts and science. Adjust your thinking about issues. Consider ways to change your ideas when necessary. Consciously improve your communication skills as this is important in both your working and personal lives. Develop your creative skills too as this will help you to face challenges that may confront you.

RECHARGE YOURSELF

We need to constantly recharge ourselves. To do this we might have to escape from reality. Make the place that you live and work beautiful. If you have a good view of nature from where you work, you will feel energized and refreshed throughout.

CULTIVATE HOBBIES

> "Today is life — the only life you are sure of.
> Make the most of today. Get interested in something.
> Shake yourself awake. Develop a hobby.
> Let the winds of enthusiasm sweep through you.
> Live today with gusto."
>
> Dale Carnegie

To have zest, have enjoyment and pleasure, consider having a hobby. There are so many activities to undertake, from collecting postcards to gardening and home improvement. Hobbies will make you a more interesting person. This is because you will have something to talk about and occupy yourself. Get involved in a task or hobby which is challenging but at the same time does not overwhelm you. Hobbies give you pleasure, fun and a sense of consistency. It helps to do work in your special areas. When you are challenged, you will experience great enjoyment. Perhaps you may wish to paint, do sculpture or pottery work.

We should also travel and enjoy the cultures and traditions of other countries. Visiting art galleries and learning to appreciate the art exhibited in these places will give us a better understanding of humanity. Going to museums and learning the history of nations and the development of various cultures will broaden our outlook on life and make us appreciate the world in which we currently live. We should develop the habit of frequenting theatres and attending plays, musicals and opera productions.

These activities will influence your creative spirits and rejuvenate and excite you. They will also provide you with much fun and pleasure. It helps to engage in the creative arts. Try your hand at painting with oils, crayons or water colours. Use other materials like metal, clay, plasticine, porcelain and create sculptures and ceramic items. Join a dance class or learn to play a musical instrument. Happy people tend to be involved in leisure activities which engage their skills. Make it a practice to engage yourself in a new activity at least once a week.

STRIVE FOR BALANCE

To feel pleasure, enthusiasm and excitement in what we do, we should ensure that we do not over-extend ourselves and overdo things. This applies to all areas of life, like eating, working, playing and drinking. Strive for a balance and then life will be enjoyable. Maintaining a balance is essential for a happy life. Likewise we need to balance the energy, time and focus that we expend on the different sectors of our life. This includes our self, our family, our friends and our career. Spending too much time and concentration on one aspect of our life will not be healthy. Practice visualization. From time to time, visualize your-self in happy situations, in perfect situations and soon you will realize these situations.

Chapter 6

PUT ZING INTO YOUR LIFE

Zing is the quality that makes you lively or interesting, of being full of energy. It can also mean to be vivacious. Having zing in your life will contribute to your general happiness. To have zing, we will first have to learn how to cope with stress and to keep active. We should practice measures that will help us to be organized so that we can avoid feeling stressed. One measure that will help us to be organized is time management. To give us energy, we should try to overcome issues, challenges and activities that cause us to feel listless and tired.

COPING WITH STRESS

"In times of great stress or adversity, it's always best to keep busy, to plow your anger and your energy into something positive."

Lee Iacocca

EFFECTS OF STRESS

Let us examine stress first. Stress is bad for the health. It causes tension and people react differently to this. Some may grind their teeth and frown all the time.

The indications of stress include overeating or in some cases not eating, increased smoking, increased drinking, lack of concentration, forgetfulness, indecisiveness, excessive worrying, mood swings, lack of coordination, difficulty working on small tasks, obsessive thoughts, keeping away from other people and neglecting one's personal appearance. Stress can also result in serious diseases, such as headaches, high blood pressure, heart attacks, anxiety, emotional problems, cancer and back pain. We cannot be happy when we are stressed to the maximum.

WHAT GENERATES STRESS?

We become stressed when our pace of work is hectic and when we over commit ourselves. Stress also occurs when we practice a lifestyle which focuses on consumerism. This type of lifestyle causes us to believe that the acquisition of wealth and material possessions will make us happy. We tell ourselves that we will be happy if and when we purchase a new item, a new product. Unfortunately, all this does is to cause us to feel stress and anxiety. Desiring a higher standard of living also causes stress.

Stress is also generated when we feel that our life is becoming more competitive, when we want the best for our children and we become overly concerned about their education and development. We experience high levels of stress when we spend far too much time worrying and being overprotective of our children and other family members. Hence, to feel happier and more content with our life, we should not worry as much or be overprotective with our children and other family members. We experience stress too when we compare ourselves with certain people. Difficult though it might be, it would be best to try to avoid making such comparisons.

Certain events which bring out change in our lives can also cause stress. These events might be a death or serious illness in the family. Divorce or separation can also result in stress among the family members. When we get married and have babies, we may also encounter stress. Likewise, when we start a new job, become redundant or when we retire, we may experience stress.

Other causes of stress might be when we are financially stretched or when we become bankrupt. Hence, a good suggestion is to watch your spending and debt incurrence and pay your bills on time. Prepare a budget and adhere to it throughout. Establish a budget for yourself so you do not overspend. In this way, you will be able to make relevant purchases. Occasionally, you should treat yourself. Either buy or do something good for yourself. Keeping to a budget and planning a schedule and timetable for yourself will ensure that you pay your bills on time.

One of the most stressful experiences we face is when we move house. It helps to remind ourselves that events are merely temporary. The stress and grievances you bear will soon fade and your life will change. What you need is time to help you cope with these events.

RESPONDING TO CHALLENGES

The way in which we respond to challenges can either make us feel happy or unhappy. The less secure person will complain and fret about his or her situation and will put the blame for the problem on others. He or she may even give up altogether. The more confident, matured person will seize the problem and look upon the problem as a learning opportunity. The problem will give him or her, the opportunity to change, to improve and to be enriched. A good example is that of Michael Jordan the Basketball player. He was not accepted in the Basketball team at 15. However, he did not give up but instead practiced continually. He was accepted in the team the next year. In Michael Jordan's case, he believed in himself and in his ability to play basketball. Not once did he give up.

When faced with challenges, we need to change some of our expectations as well as the way we do things. Only then will we be able to experience happiness even when our situation has changed. If we resist the change, we will not be as happy. However, when we have big decisions to make about ourselves and our lives, we should always consider them carefully and over time. These decisions might involve our job and career, marital status, housing situation, family size and moving to new locations. Do not make these decisions hastily.

FATIGUE AND A LACK OF SATISFACTION

"Great is the power of habit. It teaches us to bear fatigue and to despise wounds and pain."

Cicero

There are times too when we may experience a lack of satisfaction in the work that we perform and feel a lack of purpose in our jobs and our personal life. This may cause us to feel fatigued and we may not wish to see other people. When situations arise, try to handle them immediately so that they do not become difficult and ugly.

When we feel that we are missing something in our lives, we may find ourselves lacking in humour, creativity and fun. Life becomes a boring routine and we lack enthusiasm for all that is happening around us. This is when and why we need to put zing into our lives. We need to keep telling ourselves that life is great, that what we do in our jobs and our personal life is significant to many.

HANDLING A LOSS

To overcome stress and to be relaxed and happy, it helps to learn how to handle situations of loss. These involve traumatic experiences or death. If you can face the situation and recover from it, you will soon be happier. We feel sad when we expect to experience a loss. We should learn to banish unnecessary sadness from our lives.

TAKE CARE OF YOURSELF

It is important to care about yourself and to look after your own well-being. When you feel good, you will feel happy. Often, we forget to look after our own well-being. Remember to congratulate yourself for your achievements in life, be they big or small. Explore many different ways to be happy. They need not be big occasions but they could be just small moments. In this way, you you will keep happy most of the time. Some other suggestions as to what you can do to look after your well-being:

- Practice meditation every day.
- Engage in spiritual reflection.
- Go for massages and facials as they help relax the mind and body.
- Give or get yourself a manicure or pedicure.
- Sit in the sauna or steam room at your health club.
- Use the Jacuzzi and swim in the local pool.
- A good way to overcome stress is to spend a day at a spa. Indulge in a body scrub, a massage, a facial and any other treatment that the spa may provide.
- If you cannot get to a spa, then soak in bubble bath in a bath tub at home. Light some scented candles, play soft music and drink a glass of champagne.
- It helps to look good. Put on something special and make yourself look good. The compliments which you receive will make you feel good about yourself.
- Always be comfortable with your attire. Make sure that it is appropriate for the occasion that you are attending. Brightly coloured clothes will make you feel happy. Hence, plan your wardrobe.

- Ensure that your shoes are comfortable as pinched feet contribute to unhappiness.
- Put on some nice scent or cologne.
- Spend time discovering the world around you.
- Go on weekend trips for a change of scenery and just to relax.
- Try different experiences, for example, go Bungee jumping, take a roller coaster ride or try flying in a hot air balloon. Make sure though that your heart condition is ready for these unusual activities.
- Adopt as many physical activities as you can.
- Walk in parks and nature reserves so you can enjoy the natural surroundings. Look at flowers, plants and trees. Look at the way the insects, reptiles and animals behave. Admire their form and shape. Marvel at the splendour of a butter-fly. Enjoy the beauty of a single flower.
- Appreciate a puppy and be fascinated by a beetle.
- Cultivate the habit of being by yourself and enjoying your own company. In this way, you will never be lonely. Being with yourself as you walk in the park is therapeutic and it will give you more vitality.
- Your spirit will be happier when you walk in the park or botanic gardens. Stop and look at the clouds. Watch the sun set as you sit or walk on a beach. See how the moon comes up, particularly over a calm stretch of water. Watch the sunrise as well. Indulge yourself in the serenity and calm-ness of nature. Walk in the rain. Listen to the rain. All these suggested activities can be done on your own or with other people. What is good about them is that they help to gen-erate a sense of well-being. Your day then becomes special, becomes different and you will be happier.
- Plan a dinner with your spouse, loved one or friends out in the open.

- Surround yourself with warm colours like pink, rose, orange, and red as they will make you feel comfortable, warm and happy.

TAKE A VACATION

We need to take a vacation from time to time. You must learn how to take a short break from work and recognize that your absence will not cause things to come to a standstill when you are away. When we go on vacation, it means being away from our work and everyday activities. For a few days or a few weeks, we enjoy ourselves and we become happier. We can think of this for the rest of the year and it can help us to stay happy. Take a camera with you and take and keep photographs of places you visit and people you meet. This will be your pictorial biography. Try exotic food, different cuisines and bring excitement into your life.

Vacations can help to remind us of how we can try to be happy everyday. They help to remove the stress that we experience from our daily routines. When we are very involved with our work and our lives, we sometimes fail to have fun. Go on an exciting cruise or just stay home and relax as if you are at a resort. Stay by the beach and watch the waves sweep in to the beach every day. Consider eco-tourist vacations. Visit Bangkok or France for cooking classes. The change in scenery which you will experience when you stay elsewhere on vacation will help to keep you destressed and happy.

EXERCISE

"In general, any form of exercise, if pursued continuously, will help train us in perseverance."

Mao Tze-Tung

One way to keep active and to reduce stress is to exercise. Exercise will also make you a livelier person and give you lots of energy. You can then undertake all the activities that you enjoy pursuing. Besides toning your muscles and making them stronger, your overall body condition will also improve. Exercise keeps the body in peak condition. Your blood circulates and you feel great about yourself and your body. Your posture will improve and you will move quickly.

Endorphins, which have been described as the body's feel good chemical, are produced when we exercise. They give us a strong sense of well being and our mental health will improve. Exercise improves our internal sense of balance. As has been said many times before, a healthy body helps develop a healthy mind. We should therefore look after ourselves and cultivate healthy habits.

Much has been written about the advantages of aerobic exercise. It not only promotes health and energy but also helps to put off mild depression and anxiety. This is because when we exercise, our body releases natural painkillers and antidepressants such as dopamine, adrenaline/epinephrine and serotonin. Emotional problems abound with inactivity. So stay active and exercise.

It will help to promote a better self-image. Exercise will help you to be happy and to love life more. It also helps to promote and strengthen our inner core of contentment. Try exercising for half an hour three times a week as regular exercise gives us much energy. Go for a brisk walk in the morning. It is good to spend time outdoors so you can take in the fresh air. Try Pilates, Yoga or Tai Chi.

Besides exercising in the gym, there are many sports that can be pursued. Tennis, golf, hockey, cricket, netball, football, rugby, to name a few, Then there's hip-hop dancing, salsa, latin aerobics, bhangra aerobics, and line dancing. Dance to music on your own to feel the exhilaration and energy that you get from the music. Much of the tension which causes us to feel poorly can be released from our body by engaging in a regular exercise programme.

SLEEP

"True silence is the rest of the mind; it is to the spirit what sleep is to the body, nourishment and refreshment."

Sir William Penn

Exercise relaxes us and helps us to sleep better. Happy people will ensure that they make time for sleep. Get a good night's sleep. Sleep is good as it can help us cope with anxiety and depression. In turn, we will feel good and have lots of energy. People who do not get enough sleep will feel tired and this will make them less alert and unhappy. Your body, in particular your brain, needs sleep. The brain needs to relax. When we get enough sleep, we work better and we feel good at the end of the day. It has been documented that the quality and quantity of sleep affects our health, well-being and our positive outlook. With good sleep and a healthy lifestyle, you will wake up each morning feeling good and your day will be filled with much fun and success.

GET SOME REST

Adopt a relaxed, calm and healthy lifestyle. We need to build into our lives specific periods of rest as this will help us to be more alert. If you feel lethargic take five deep, slow breaths. This will help to increase your energy levels and boost your moods. When we are physically and mentally rested, we become more productive, more creative and more efficient. We can solve problems better and make creative decisions. We are also emotionally satisfied and are less prone to anger and irritation. In short, we are happier.

DIET

To adopt a healthy lifestyle, be aware of the right diet to adopt and the practices to implement so as to prevent the onset of certain illnesses. We need to be careful with the food that we consume when we are eating out. Consuming some fruit every day is desirable as it contributes towards your well-being. Not only will you feel better about yourself but you will also feel capable and happier with your life. As the old adage states, "*eat an apple a day to keep the doctor away.*" Make fresh fruit juices and smoothies in the morning with a blender or juicer. Taking this in the morning will help you to feel energized and happy. Take vitamins. Drink lots of water so you will have much energy. Dehydration can make you feel low and irritable.

Eating the right foods will contribute to your inner sense of balance and emotional well-being. Fruits, vegetables and fish are good to consume. Avoid fatty foods. The right diet will help you to feel more content and happier with life. Do not skip meals or over eat as this will cause mood swings. Some people like to use herbs to promote happiness.

MEDICAL CARE

It helps to learn how to manage pain. Take note of your health and have regular check ups with your doctor. Keep to one family physician throughout so that the doctor has a good understanding of your health situation and is better able to advise and treat you. Health problems can drain you of your energy very quickly.

MUSIC AND SINGING

"Without music, life would be a mistake."

Nietzsche

88

Music has a good effect on the emotions. Listen to uplifting music. Music stimulates the brain. It gives us much excitement and happiness. Boredom can cause you to be distressed.

Singing is a good way to feel happy. Many of us like to listen to music and very often we sing along with the music which we hear in the background. The Japanese introduced karaoke as a way to get people to destress themselves. Karaoke has since caught on and is very popular throughout the world. According to native American Indians, singing can give you much happiness. When we sing out loud, with expression and with emotion, we release our feelings and we become less introverted and unhappy about ourselves. When we sing, we are also energized. Listeners are similarly energized.

When we sing or when we listen to others sing, we often feel like dancing and we start to tap our feet. This makes us feel happy. There may be some songs which make you feel good and well prepared to face the challenges in this world. Try to find the lyrics to these songs. Then sing them whenever you feel unhappy and they will make you feel better. Try whistling a happy tune instead of singing. Sing when you feel unhappy. Try doing this when you are in the shower and picture the water washing away your problems and your unhappiness. Sing for the sheer joy of it.

TIME MANAGEMENT

"Lost wealth may be replaced by industry, lost knowledge by study, lost health by temperance or medicine, but lost time is gone forever."

Samuel Smiles

Be careful with your time and learn to time manage effectively. Some suggested ways to do this:

- Prioritize your tasks.
- Compile a list of things to do.

- Work systematically to achieve what is on the list.
- Complete one task first before commencing work on the next task. In this way, you can concentrate well on the next task and apply the appropriate energy and time on it. You will also feel happier and satisfied that you have completed the first task.
- When working on a new task, spend a bit of time at the beginning to understand what is required and how to complete the task.
- Spend time working on the task so that you complete it well. In this way you avoid having to correct errors and redoing the task later. This will only make you feel unhappy.
- To avoid procrastinating on difficult tasks, decide to work on these first.
- Difficult tasks are best worked on early in the day as your energy and motivation levels are higher then. Organizing your tasks in this way will enable you to complete more work more quickly. This will motivate you to perform more and better work.
- Do not work till late into the night as this will make you tired the next day.
- Plan some time at the end of each day to help you to relax after a day's work. This will help to reenergize you as well.
- Set yourself some goals for the day.
- Keep to your appointments and maintain punctuality.

If you plan your time effectively, you will not need to rush around and be stressed as a result. Trying to meet deadlines without giving yourself sufficient time is also stressful. When a situation arises and you are unable to meet someone, attend a meeting or change a programme make sure that you let the people concerned know so that they are not left waiting for you. While they will be pleased for having been informed of your absence or of the change in your programme they will also feel happier with the arrangement. In this way too people will recognize that you are responsible and dependable. You will feel good about yourself.

OTHER ACTIVITIES

To keep active and to be happy, we should not spend too much time as a couch potato and try to watch less television. Time spent viewing television could be better spent on other activities. We could learn to communicate better with others, engage in happy activities with our family members and friends, exercise, sign up for classes, dance and engage in interesting hobbies. Cultivate common interests with your family and friends. This will help to strengthen your relationship with them. Never stop learning and adapting.

Read extensively as reading helps you to learn as well as keeps you entertained. You will feel happy and satisfied. Most people are happier engaged in a leisure activity like gardening or scuba diving rather than watching television. Watching the news on television and documentaries which focus on warfare, health problems and tension will only upset you and make you feel unhappy. Instead, it would be far better to view programmes which emphasize the good and optimistic things in life and which are positive and upbeat.

PHYSICAL ACTIVITY

Physical activity like cleaning, cooking and gardening can help to improve your moods and feelings. If you like gardening, then try planting flowers and even keeping a vegetable and herb garden. Together with the act of pulling weeds and making a garden, terrace or patio look good, gardening can make things happier for you generally.

PETS

"If you pick up a starving dog and make him prosperous,
he will not bite you."

Mark Twain

Keep a pet as pets can bring you much happiness. The closer you get to your pet, the greater pleasure you will experience. Pets can provide you with warmth and love. It has been said that people who keep pets tend to live longer and happier lives.

MOTIVATIONAL MATERIALS

When you feel miserable, read books that will motivate and inspire you to change or those that will guide and help you feel better. Try listening to audio recordings and attend personal development workshops. Read books written by inspirational people. Listen and talk to them when they present talks or conduct workshops. It helps to accept the advice of people who are more experienced. Read the latest motivational books as you may acquire some new and timely suggestions.

We all have a quest for inspiration to help us achieve excellence in all that we undertake, to make progress everyday and to overcome troubles, tough times and difficulties. Be inspired by happy people. The inspiration and encouragement that we get from all this will put us in good stead. Learn to meditate and engage in visualizations and affirmations.

KEEP BUSY AND REMOVE CLUTTER

Keep yourself busy as we tend to feel happy when we have much to do as compared to when we do not have anything with which to occupy our time. Keep active and feel invigorated by throwing out the clutter in your life. First, look at the junk that you may have accumulated over time. Give away what you do not need and those things which you no longer use. When you give things away, you create space so that if you do purchase or obtain new items there is space for you to place them.

The Chinese art of Feng Shui maintains that old piled up stuff will not make you feel good. Once you remove the clutter, energy will be released into the environment and you will feel happier. To help avoid filling your home with clutter, only purchase items which are important to you. In this way too, you will enjoy the items and appreciate them better.

EMOTIONAL BAGGAGE

Just as we handle physical things, we should also learn to throw away the junk in our emotional life. Do not harbour grudges and carry emotional baggage with you. It will drain you of all energy instead. Life for you then will have no zing in it. Learn to forgive others. Learn to forgive yourself. Do not blame yourself all the time.

Avoid allowing frustrations and disappointments to cloud your peace of mind. Learn to distinguish between what is important and what is not important. When you are faced with something that is emotionally upsetting, ask yourself if it is worth getting distressed about it. If you do this often enough, you will soon realize that most things which you would worry about are truly not worth losing any sleep over. Do not erode your energy by throwing temper tantrums, worrying and grudging others.

WORRY

"Do not anticipate trouble, or worry about what may never happen. Keep in the sunlight."

Benjamin Franklin

When you start brooding, you can soon be depressed and anti-social. Eventually, you will avoid doing things for yourself, neglect your family and not be able to serve the community and society. Worrying then is not to be encouraged. Learn to free your mind from worry. Avoid anticipating things. Instead, handle each crisis that comes to you one at a time.

Do not worry unnecessarily. Keep a small notebook with you at all times and record your worries and concerns in the book. Address these worries and concerns later. We often worry when we maintain very high standards for ourselves and we feel that we cannot match these standards. Hence, we need to set realistic standards for ourselves. Sometimes, we believe that we do not deserve any happiness ourselves especially when we are angry with ourselves for not getting things right. We therefore have to learn to forgive ourselves for our mistakes.

We should not waste time and energy worrying about things which have happened. Avoid thinking of how your life would have been if you had made another decision or had changed things. You will just end up feeling unhappy. When you feel anxious, worried and depressed, try sleeping as sleep is a good remedy. Try a change in routine too as this can help to liven you a little.

"What's the use of worrying?
It never was worthwhile,
So pack up your troubles in your old kit bag,
And smile, smile, smile."

AVOID WASTING YOUR ENERGY

To avoid wasting energy and to channel your energy into productive activities, there are some things that you should practice and some things that you can avoid doing. Do not bother to look at junk mail. Delete anything that looks like junk mail from your inbox on your computer. If it is printed junk mail, just discard it immediately. If you get too many phone calls which take up your time, you could try placing an answering machine to screen your calls. If when you make a call and you are put on hold, decide if it is worth waiting or if it might be better to just ring off. If you decide to wait, try to do something as you wait to make use of the time profitably.

When helping other people to solve their problems, try to establish a balance. Do not get too involved as this can drain you of all energy. It can make you feel listless and tired. The same applies to family issues. If you get too involved with these problems, you will not have enough strength to do much else.

BE ORGANISED

To have zing in our life, we need to be more organized in the way that we live our life. For example, to avoid forgetting about birthdays and anniversaries, we could keep a record either on the computer or in a book. To avoid wasting time looking for the right gifts to buy, the wrapping paper and cards to buy, we could buy gifts, paper and cards ahead of time. Sometimes, it is cheaper too to buy during sale periods, when you are overseas or when you see something advertised in a catalogue.

Design a routine for the work that you undertake, be it in the house or elsewhere. This will stop you from worrying as to what to do next. If you are not organized in this way, you will be stressed and then you will not be able to complete all the work that you have to do each day. Being organized contributes to your happiness. You can then avoid having to experience problems and of encountering crisis after crisis.

BIBLIOGRAPHY

BOOKS

Baird, D (2000). *A Thousand Paths to Happiness*. Naperville, IL: MQ Publications Limited.

De Bono, E (1977). *The Happiness Purpose*. England: Penguin Books.

De Vries, MK (2000). *The Happiness Equation*. London: Vermillion.

Foster, R and Hicks, G (1999). *How We Choose To Be Happy*. New York: The Berkley Publishing Group.

Freeman, WB (2000). *If I Really Wanted To Be Happy, I Would*. Oklahoma: Concepts, Inc, Honor Books.

Gore, A (1998). *You Can Be Happy*. Australia: Prentice Hall.

Hampton, T and Harper, R (1999). *99 Ways To Be Much Happier Every Day*. Gretna: Pelican Publishing Company.

Happiness (2000). Surrey, England: Four Seasons Publishing.

Hayries, C (1998). *2002 Ways To Cheer Yourself Up*. Kansas City: Andrews McMeel Publishing.

Hoggard, L (2005). *How to be Happy*. London: BBC Books.

Layard, R (2005). *Happiness Lessons from a New Science*. USA: The Penguin Press.

Lykken, D (1999). *Happiness*. New York: St Martin's Griffin.

Matthews, A (1999). *Happiness In A Nutshell*. Australia: Seashell Publishers.

Niven, D (2000). *The 100 Simple Secrets of Happy People*. New York: Harper.

Oliver, JD (2005). *Happiness: How to Find it and Keep It*. London: Duncan Baird Publishers.

Peiffer, V (2002). *Inner Happiness: Positive Steps to Feeling Complete*. London: Judy Piatkus (Publishers) Ltd.

Post, S and Peacock, O (1995). *What Is Happiness?* Illinois: Successories Publishing.

Prager, D (1998). *Happiness is a Serious Problem.* New York: HarperCollins Publishers, Inc.

Prentiss, C (2000). *The Little Book of Secrets, Vol 1.* California, USA: Power Press.

Ricard, M (2007). *Happiness: A Guide to Developing Life's Most Important Skill.* London: Atlantic Books.

Shea, S.C (2004). *Happiness Is.: Unexpected Answers to Practical Questions In Curious Times.* Deerfield Beach, Florida: Health Communications, Inc.

Summers, H and Watson, A (2006). *The Book of Happiness.* West Sussex: Capstone Publishing Limited.

Webber, C (2000). *Get The Happiness Habit.* Illinois, USA: NTC Publishing Group.

Were, K (1999). *Help Yourself to Happiness.* Melbourne: Thomas Lothian Pty Ltd.

WEBSITES

Bronstein, H (1991). *Happiness.* Retrieved October 6, 2005 from www.30goodminutes.org

Csikszentmihalyi, M (2005). *The Secrets of Happiness:* Retrieved October 7, 2005 from www.timesonline.co.uk

Emmett, T (2005). *What is Happiness?* Retrieved October 10, 2005 from www.ezinearticles.com

Fordyce, M (2005). *What is Happiness?* Retrieved October 5, 2005 from www.thehappinessshow.com

Hamrick, JR (2005). *Choosing Joy: Why and How.* Retrieved October 10, from www.ezinearticles.com

Heij, A (2001). *Happiness is a Decision.* Retrieved October 10, 2005 from *www.reamagick.com*

Heylighen, F (1999). *Happiness:* Retrieved October 7, 2005 from www.pcp.lanl.gov

Kenner, E (2005). *What is Happiness?* Retrieved October 5, 2005 from www.drkenner.com

Ketchian, L (2003). *Be Happy Zone.* Retrieved October 5, 2005 from www.happinessclub.com

Khanna, R (1996). *How to be a Winner in the Game of Happiness.* Retrieved October 7, 2005 from www.lifepositive.com

Knapp, S (2005). *Are You Really Happy?* Retrieved October 7, 2005 from www.stephen-knapp.com

Leonhardt, D (2005). *What is the Definition of Happiness Anyway?* Retrieved October 5, 2005 from www.thehappy guy.com

Myers, DG (2005). *Suggestions for a Happier Life.* Retrieved October 6, 2005 from www.davidmyers.org

Myers, DG (2004). *The Secret to Happiness.* Retrieved October 6, 2005 from www.yesmagazine.org

Ritchie, B (2005). *10 Ways To Put Sunshine In Your Day.* Retrieved October 10, 2005 from www.ezinearticles.com

Russell, P (2005). *Happiness — The Mind's Bottom Line.* Retrieved October 10, 2005 from www.peterussell.com

Tavris, C (2005). *Happy?* Retrieved October 6, 2005 from www.the-tls.co.uk

Varughese, S (2005). Seven Steps to Happiness. Retrieved on October 7, 2005 from www.lifepositive.com

Vickers, E (2002). *On Happiness.* Retrieved October 7, 2005 from www.museumofconceptualart.com

Warter, C (1999). *Happiness is Your Birthright.* Retrieved October 7, 2005 from www.newtimes.org

Weinberg, N (2000). *The Secret of Happiness.* Retrieved October 7, 2005 from www.aish.com

Wong, T.P (2003). *Finding Happiness Through Suffering.* Retrieved October 7, 2005 from www.meaning.ca

NEWSPAPER AND MAGAZINE ARTICLES

Happiness is Being Helpful. *Birmingham Mail*, 1 June 2006.

Bone, A. The Secret of Happiness. *NZ Listener*, 18 March 2006.

Boniwell, I. The Undervalued Component of Happiness. *BBC News Online*, 10 May 2006.

Curry, M. Nelson's Guide to Happiness: Keep Laughing. *Associated Press Newswires*, 20 May 2006.

Easton, M. The Politics of Happiness, *BBC News Online*, 23 May 2006.

Strike a Happy Balance, *Evening Express*, 28 March 2006.

Follis, D. Reasonable Happiness is All We Can Expect. *The News Gazette*, 17 March 2006.

Hayden, G. Pursuit of Happiness. *Mind Your Body*, 28 February 2007.

Hise, P. The Key to Happiness: The Old Fashioned Golden Rule. *The Richmond Times Dispatch*, 28 May 2006.

Jeevan, S. Happiness Lies Here and Now. *The Hindu*, 22 May 2006.

Harrell, E. Money Really Can't Buy You Happiness, Poll Confirms. *The Scotsman*, 3 May 2006.

Extra Income No Longer Generates Extra Happiness in Society. *Hindustan Times*, 3 May 2006.

Kearns, M. Happiness in the Workplace is … a Thing of Sheer Beauty. *Irish Independent*, 29 March 2006.

Kerevan, G. Word of the Week: Happiness. *The Scotsman*, 6 May 2006.

Lloyd, J. The Economics of Happiness. *The Sunday Times*, 7 May 2006.

Marsden, S. Money Really Can't Buy Happiness. *Press Association Newswire*, 3 May 2006.

PG&E Troubleshooter Finds Happiness in Helping People. *Merced Sun-Star*, 15 May 2006.

Rudin, M. Is there a Happiness Formula? *BBC News Online*, 2 June 2006.

How Volunteering Brings Happiness. *Sevenoaks Chronicle*, 1 June 2006.

Skinner, J. Have We Lost Formula for Happiness? *Western Daily Press*, 9 May 2006.

Stewart, D. What Happiness Means To Me. *Irish Independent*, 3 May 2006.

Singaporeans the Least Happy People in Asia. *The Straits Times*, 13 July 2006.

Don't worry, Be Happy, Say MPs. *The Straits Times*, 11 November 2006.

Don't Worry, Be Happy. *The Straits Times*, 25 August 2007.

PM Lee's New Year Message of Happiness. *Today*, 28 January 2006.

The Happy Issue. *Weekend Today*, 28–29 January 2006.

Womack, S. Happiness Levels are on the Slide, Finds Poll. *The Daily Telegraph*, 3 May 2006.

Zaslow, J. The Secrets of Happiness: Emerging Field Explores What Causes Joyful Emotions. *Pittsburgh Post-Gazette*, 5 April 2006.

INDEX

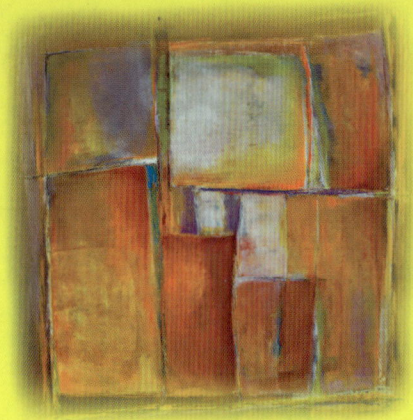

Zany, zeal, zest and Zing.
the Z Way to Happiness

Written in a pragmatic, yet inspirational style, this book provides relevant and useful information on happiness. It includes a brief history of happiness and motivates readers to apply strategies related to happiness in their day-to-day life. It also discusses the benefits of being happy and the consequences of being unhappy. The strategies are listed under the headings — Zany, Zeal, Zest and Zing. Each chapter is unique and will be of great interest to readers.

Key Features

- Contains pragmatic and easy-to-implement strategies to live a happy life
- Provides a comprehensive review of views of different writers and philosophers on happiness
- Includes a description of happiness and explains the benefits of being happy

World Scientific
www.worldscientific.com

6765 sc

ISBN-13 978-981-279-350-8(pbk)
ISBN-10 981-279-350-X(pbk)

9 789812 793508